REFLEX ZONE THERAPY OF THE FEET

A therapist's guide to this subtle method of compression massage, including reflex zones of the nervous system, causal reflex zones and case histories.

REFLEX ZONE THERAPY OF THE FEET

A Textbook for Therapists

by

HANNE MARQUARDT

Introduction by Dr Erich Rauch

Translated from the German by
Ann Callard Lett

THORSONS PUBLISHERS INC.
New York

Thorsons Publishers Inc.
377 Park Avenue South
New York, New York 10016

First U.S. Edition 1984

LIBRARY OF CONGRESS CATALOGING IN PUBLICATION DATA

Marquardt, Hanne.
  Reflex zone therapy of the feet.

  Translation of: Reflexzonenarbeit am Fuss.
  Bibliography: p.
  Includes index.
  1. Reflexotherapy.   2. Foot.   I. Title. [DNLM:
1. Reflexotherapy.   2. Foot.   WB 962 M357r]
RM723.R43M3713   1984   617.8'22   84-2455
ISBN 0-7225-0791-7 (pbk.)

Printed in Hong Kong by South China Printing Co.

Thorsons Publishers Inc. are distributed to the trade by
Inner Traditions International Ltd., New York

CONTENTS

Translator's Note and Preface to the First English Edition

This is the first authoritative manual on Reflex Zone Therapy of the Feet to come into English print since Eunice Ingham's books, *Stories the Feet Can Tell* and *Stories the Feet Have Told* were published forty years ago. A very great deal has been added to our knowledge of the subject since that time through the work done by Mrs Marquardt and her colleagues.

Several of the treatments mentioned in this book are better known on the Continent than they are in some English-speaking countries. However, a growing interest in alternative medicine, and the reassessment of what is practical and useful in allopathic medicine, as well as the part which can be fulfilled by some traditional and less well known methods, is already well under way. Those who care for the sick are under a continuing obligation to look anew at ways of alleviating pain and disability for their patients.

After twenty-five years as nurse, midwife, ward sister and tutor in England and South Africa, I became aquainted with Reflex Zone Therapy of the Feet after a serious personal accident, and subsequently attended the Introductory and Advanced courses at Mrs Marquardt's School in Germany. Courses are now being held in the United Kingdom, and it is hoped that with the publication of this book more people will come to know something of this interesting and valuable work.

Reflex Zone Therapy is not a panacea for all ills. In its practice the practitioner requires disciplined application to become skilled so that the best results may be obtained. but the field in which it can be put to use is wide and, practised well, it will assist many people.

This book is a translation. I have tried to convey the ideas and explanations given by Mrs Marquardt in a form that will be understood and received by a lay and professional English-speaking public. Any errors of interpretation must be mine alone, yet I trust that the book is true to the spirit and practice of Reflex Zone Therapy as taught by Mrs Marquardt.

ANN CALLARD LETT
Principal: British School of Reflex Zone Therapy of the Feet
25 Brooks Mews
London W1
England

Foreword

I was introduced to Reflex Zone Therapy of the Feet through reading Eunice Ingham's original book *Stories the Feet Can Tell* in 1965. My interest was sufficiently roused to pursue the subject further, and my colleagues and I began to examine the feet of most of our patients and, where it seemed appropriate, to treat them. After hundreds of such cases there remained no doubt in our minds that the accounts given by Mrs Ingham, and the discoveries made by Dr William Fitzgerald were factual, impartial, verifiable and medically sound, and not illusory.

Numerous areas of the feet lie in a particular reflex relationship and connection to identifiable zones of the body and its organs. This is a help in both diagnosis and treatment, as can readily be proven. The feet, seldom submitted to therapy, usually fitted into tight shoes, and rarely exposed to the air, may now, thanks to Dr Fitzgerald and Mrs Ingham, become the effective starting point for the treatment of innumerable conditions.

Understandably, many of our patients were initially sceptical and even bewildered when we began to massage their feet. Those who saw no connection between their ailments and treatment of their feet were particularly perplexed.

Today, due to the renaissance of interest in acupuncture, there is a growing readiness to believe that inter-relationships exist between certain points of the body and organs widely removed from such points. Due to the wide lay acceptance of acupuncture, a similar relationship between certain areas of the feet and organs lying at some distance from these areas is now at least open to question. The concomitant feelings of 'sensitivity and well-being' which pervade the whole body in accompaniment to a massage of the reflex zones of the feet, and its undoubted therapeutic efficacy have been instrumental in bringing about this change in a short space of time.

At this stage we first learned that courses of instruction in Reflex Zone Therapy of the Feet were being held, and Mrs Hanne Marquardt, the author of this book, who had learned the method from Mrs Ingham and made it her speciality, invited us to one of these. This introductory course was most instructive. It proved again how little manual dexterity could be learned from a book alone, and brought into view the breadth and scope of the practice, and its wide range of application. Results showed themselves soon afterwards in a remarkable improvement in therapeutic effect. It was thus small wonder that Reflex Zone Therapy of the Feet established for itself a wholly scientific place amongst those of us studying holistic medicine.

In particular, Mrs Marquardt proved the value of treatment of the feet for such a wide range of ailments that it has since become a quite indispensable form of treatment amongst us. These include: disorders of the musculo-skeletal system and the spine; functional disorders of the respiratory and genito-urinary systems; developmental disorders of childhood, and several others. Many rare conditions are amenable to treatment with this method provided that their reflex signature has been visibly and palpably engraved on the relevant foot zone.

Our combined experience in this field has left us in no doubt that a method as effective as this requires that those who wish to practise should have the necessary basic knowledge, and sufficient practical and theoretical training. Mrs Marquardt, in every sense the fit and proper person to train pupils in this discipline, strongly recommends several training courses. Aspiring practitioners should nevertheless have had some previous training and experience in working with the sick, either in nursing, physiotherapy, or some related discipline, and they should have undergone a series of reflex zone massages of the feet.

Despite the merits of this form of treatment, it is possible to introduce errors into its practice A therapist working without due care will bring to the patient a less effective form of treatment, and disrepute upon the method. One can only be warned against those who set up training courses without relevant experience. Those who would truly learn must shun bad teachers. The many mechanical aids which have appeared in recent times and have been widely promoted must also be avoided. There is no fundamental justification for the claims made on their behalf, nor do they satisfy any medical criteria. They do not permit the right application of pressure or the right touch.

A prerequisite for this work is a good working relationship with a doctor, at best with one who has an understanding of the subject. Therein lie the interests of the patient, the therapist, and not least of all, the method.

Finally, it must be said that amongst all the medical sciences there is not one form of therapy which does not have its boundaries. Reflex Zone Therapy of the Feet is no exception. It should not be practised indiscriminately, nor with all one's critical faculties suspended. Its practice must be governed by awareness of its scope and limitations. It is irresponsible and unethical to raise false hopes.

We find the evaluation of abnormal findings in the feet particularly important. It matters not whether they are recognized through means of sight, touch, or painful reactions which they may provoke in the patient. There are four possible causes to be considered when these abnormal findings are encountered:

1. Temporary functional overload of the organ related to that zone, e.g. in the heart zone immediately after a severe heart attack; the liver after a fatty meal; the zones relating to the eyes after a long car journey, watching television, etc.

2. Slight or insignificant dysfunction of an organ. Current clinical tests cannot as yet assess with accuracy such damage. This is referred to as damage to the tissues which has not yet become consciously or clinically manifest. The diagnostic techniques of Dr F.X. Mayr, such as electro-acupuncture, impulse dermography, etc. need to be brought into wider use in conjunction with this therapy to provide a more accurate diagnosis of such dysfunction.

3. Functional disease of the organ related to that zone.

4. Systemic disease involving that organ.

Abnormal reflex zones should not therefore be interpreted as indicating disease, nor provide the basis for making an 'interesting diagnosis'. Diagnosis is the prerogative of the doctor. When a doctor is familiar with this method he will certainly take into account diagnostic indications arising from abnormal zones on the feet, and will find them a worthy adjunct in drawing up a differential diagnosis.

There is often a great temptation to lay too much emphasis on the abnormal reflex zones found, particularly when the patient asks what this or that painful area signifies. A good practitioner, whose sole interest is the patient's progress, will only allude to the possibility of malfunction of organs or systems in that zone, and not declare the presence of specific disease. The therapist will not therefore create anxiety or a neurotic response in a patient who has a hypochondriacal tendency.

Above all else, *Nil Nocere!* — Do No Harm — remains the maxim of all healing disciplines. I direct all those who wish to practise Reflex Zone Massage of the Feet to reflect on this statement, and to base their work upon it.

The publication of this book has met a great need. The writer, Mrs Hanne Marquardt, has given within its covers expression to all the results of her training in this speciality arising from her knowledge and practical experience. She has laid the necessary foundation for all who are interested in the practice of Reflex Zone Therapy of the Feet. The practical knowledge which she has acquired, and her dedicated concern over the years have led to Reflex Zone Massage of the Feet gaining its properly recognized place alongside other manual therapies. The many Do-it-Yourself methods which have developed recently are something of a threat to this recognition. When the therapist truly endeavours to understand all that is embraced in this method, both therapist and patient will find joy in its practice, and unanticipated success will often be the result.

I hope that this book finds a wide audience, and wish for the author and her numerous readers and pupils, much success.

Dr Erich Rauch
A-9082 Maria Worth/Karnetern
W. Germany

BUSINESS REPLY CARD

FIRST CLASS   PERMIT NO. 5   LIVINGSTON, MT

POSTAGE WILL BE PAID BY ADDRESSEE

SUMMIT UNIVERSITY PRESS
Box A
Livingston, MT 59047-9977

We would very much appreciate having your comments on this book

Title: _____

(Please print title of book on the above line)

WE HOPE THAT YOU HAVE ENJOYED THIS BOOK AND THAT IT WILL OCCUPY A SPECIAL PLACE IN YOUR LIBRARY. IT WOULD BE HELPFUL TO US IN MEETING THE SPIRITUAL NEEDS OF OUR READERS IF YOU WILL FILL OUT AND MAIL THIS POSTAGE-FREE CARD TO US.

Your comments: _____

_____

How did this book come to your attention? _____

Your business or profession: _____

What subjects would interest you most in future publications? _____

_____

WOULD YOU CARE TO RECEIVE A FREE CATALOG OF OUR NEW PUBLICATIONS?   YES ☐   NO ☐

Mr./Mrs./Miss _____

Address _____

City/State/Zip _____

SUBSCRIBE TODAY TO THE COMING REVOLUTION: THE MAGAZINE FOR HIGHER CONSCIOUSNESS. U.S.A. $12.00 PPD. (4 ISSUES); CANADA & INTERNATIONAL $14.50 PPD.

Printed in the U.S.A.

Introduction

In the summer of 1958, whilst working as a masseuse in a sanatorium in southern Germany, I discovered a book called *Stories the Feet Can Tell*, written by Eunice Ingham in 1938. More from a sense of curiosity towards an unknown subject than out of a spirit of scientific investigation, I began to try out this unusual method of treatment. I took every available foot into my hands, palpated, observed, massaged and compared them, until I was myself persuaded that the feet represented a central switchboard, from where — I knew not how or why — observable effects over the whole of the body could be provoked.

What had begun as a non-serious curiosity in my spare time then gave place to a serious preoccupation. The therapeutic results of my massages to the feet, amateurish as they then were, encouraged me and surprised my patients. After nine years of being engrossed with the reflex zones of the feet, I finally came to meet and work with Mrs Eunice Ingham, then already eighty years old, but full of vitality, and moreover, a percipient masseuse in the U.S.A. (Sadly, she died in December 1974).

My earlier training as a nurse in England served me well, as it gave me the background knowledge and understanding of the language which I needed. This thoroughly useful and worthwhile beginning stimulated me to think continually about the development of the method, and at the same time I began to approach other interested and professional specialists. An experimental first training course in Reflex Zone Therapy of the Feet was embarked upon despite the difficulties of:

(a)   Transposing a method from the land of 'limitless

opportunities' to Europe, with its more cautious outlook;

(b) Adapting to modern needs a method of treatment whose meaning had been grasped at the beginning of the twentieth century, and which claimed to alleviate a diversity of illnesses; and . . .

(c) Explaining this form of treatment, which was as yet not understood scientifically. It had, however, been developed, refined and expanded to such a degree that it could now be taught to experienced manualtherapists.

The venture prospered. After this first attempt, numerous courses of instruction took place over the subsequent years. There have been invitations from medical professional circles to lecture and instruct in Austria, Switzerland, England, South Africa and Israel.

Meanwhile, qualified students who have attended courses in Reflex Zone Therapy of the Feet are working in twenty-six countries in Europe and abroad. In 1972 a branch school was started in Denmark for the Scandinavian countries. The ground was prepared for an English speaking subsidiary school in Johannesburg, South Africa in 1975, and affiliated schools now exist in Britain and Israel. Several large hospitals are discovering the potential of this method, and proving through experience the value of Reflex Zone Therapy of the Feet. W. Froneberg, who is particularly interested in manual therapies relating to the nervous system, stimulated by experience gained during these courses, showed that there are reflex zones relating to central and autonomic nervous systems in the feet; and he is working closely with the school here to further elucidate and expand our knowledge.

This book is the result of fruitful work done by my therapists and patients. Over the years it has become evident that an account of knowledge which has been handed down and all newly acquired information should be amalgamated in book form.

In the years to come I wish for Reflex Zone Therapy of the Feet the same vitality in its total growth as has been evident until now. I wish to pass on with faith and gratitude all that I know and have learned as a result of my experiences to 'faithful hands' to further this knowledge and work.

HANNE MARQUARDT
D-7744 Konigsfeld-Burgberg
W. Germany

NOTE TO SECOND EDITION

A revised second edition of this book has fortunately become necessary. The principal addition is information about the reflex zones to the motor part of the nervous system, which has been added by Walter Froneberg, who also contributed to the previous edition.

NOTE TO THE TENTH EDITION

After three years the tenth, completely revised edition of this book has been prepared. The reader will find several new chapters and updated, coloured diagrams. For these I thank my publishers, Karl F. Haug.

Some of the great improvements in this edition will be recognized by workers in this field. Due to her expert understanding of the human *gestalt* and its movements, Margaret Lehro has given a new impetus to the meaning of the grip sequence (the α and Ω) and its practice. It is comprehensively dealt with in the section on 'The Grip Sequence as the Foundation of this Work'. I wish to record my thanks to her.

SECTION I

1.

THE HISTORY OF REFLEX ZONE THERAPY

Dr William Fitzgerald, the founder of Zone Therapy, was born in Middletown, U.S.A. in 1872. He graduated in medicine from the University of Vermont in 1895, and then spent some years in hospitals in Vienna, Paris and London. He later practised in the Hospital for Diseases of the Ear, Nose and Throat in Hartford, Connecticut, then transferred his practice and teaching to New York, and died in Stamford, U.S.A. in 1942.

Developing the work of Dr H. Bressler, Dr Fitzgerald came to Vienna in the early years of this century to consider the possibility of treating organs through pressure points. In his book *Zone Therapy*[18] he makes some interesting remarks about its history:

> A form of treatment by means of pressure points was known in India and China 5000 years ago. This knowledge appears however to have been lost or forgotten. Perhaps it was set aside in favour of acupuncture, which emerged as the stronger growth from the same root.

In central European countries similar methods were described in 1582 by Dr Adamus and Dr A'Tatis. At about the same time Dr Ball of Leipzig published a manuscript on the treatment of separate organs of the body by means of pressure points. The great Florentine sculptor, Cellini (1500–1571), used strong pressure on his fingers and toes to relieve pain anywhere in his body, with remarkable success.

The twentieth American President, W. Garfield (1831–1881), was able to alleviate the pains he had following an assassination attempt by applying pressure to various points in his feet. No other pain-killing medicines gave him relief.

The relationship betwen reflex points and the internal organs of the body was known by various North American Indian tribes and used in the treatment of disease. This knowledge has been preserved over many centuries, and is still used in Indian reservations for the relief of pain.

Evidently, sick people — at least in Europe, Asia and America — have intuitively discovered numerous points where pressure could be applied to bring about certain known effects on other parts of the body, and have used them in the relief of their diseases. Those who today invoke the involuntary gestures of biting their teeth together, clenching their fists, or spontaneously applying pressure to an acutely painful area may well be employing relics of a similar background.

In 1916, Dr Edwin F. Bowers first publicly described the treatment propounded by Dr Fitzgerald, and called it 'Zone Therapy'. One year later their combined work appeared in the book *Zone Therapy*[19]. It contained therapeutic proposals and recommendations for doctors, dentists, gynaecologists, E.N.T. specialists and chiropractors. According to Dr George Starr White in 1925, 'the fact that today Zone Therapy is probably known more widely throughout the United States and all places where magazines and newspapers are printed than any other single method of therapy, proves that the foundation of this work is solid.'

Dr Fitzgerald gave courses of instruction and gathered about him a circle of practitioners. Diagrams of the zones of the feet and the corresponding division of the ten zones of the body appeared in the first edition of his book. He was not to know that he was thereby handing on Indian folk medicine, and giving it scientific respectability.

The groundwork had thus been laid when the American masseuse, Eunice Ingham, started her training in this discipline. She spent years gaining insight into the manner of its working. The diagrams and accounts of those around her, allied to her own practical observation, served to form the basis for her 'pressure massage' to the feet. As a result of this wide experience, Eunice Ingham played her part in putting Reflex Zone Therapy on 'its feet', concentrating her attention and knowledge on the *small surfaces* of the foot.

She developed a special, subtle method of massage, which she called the Ingham method of compression massage, described in her book *Stories the Feet Can Tell*[4, 5]. Her original massage, 'as though one was refining sugar crystals in one's hand' was continually being altered and improved during her many years of practice, and is now taught as the corner-stone of this work, at our present state of knowledge.

Between 1958 and 1967, Reflex Zone Therapy was used with success in my own practice, and since 1967 each new development has been tested in the School for Reflex Zone Therapy by fully qualified trained workers from all medical and therapeutic professions.

Thus, the method has behind it, as do many others, a gradual development. Through many centuries it has passed from being an old, intuitive folk medicine to its present adaptable form of manual therapy, by means of which the present generation can be helped.

2.
THE ZONE GRID

The practice of Reflex Zone Massage to the Feet is derived from two basic concepts:

(i)   The division of the body into *ten vertical zones*, postulated by Dr William Fitzgerald.

(ii) The corresponding *ten zone grid of the feet*, in which are dovetailed the *reflex zones*, which have been empirically known for centuries.

The Zones of the Body

The ten vertical body zones
The body is divided into ten equal, vertical zones, in which are incorporated all the organs of the head and trunk, by imaginary lines which are drawn through the head, arms, trunk and feet. There are hypotheses that these vertical fields depict stylized and simplified meridians. This interpretation, and the co-ordination of these fields, is mentioned in the early American writings.

This vertical division of the body is useful to us for work on the reflex zones of the feet, as it provides an anatomical-topographical aid, such as that used to divide the globe by meridians.

The three transverse body zones
As the ten vertical zones only allow us to locate the organs of the body in their longitudinal relationship to one another, we came in 1970 to realize as a result of our studies in the School that these vertical lines could be transected by similarly imagined

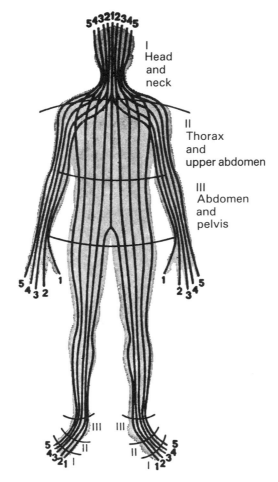

Diagram 1: Zones of the Body

transverse or horizontal lines which divide the body into transverse zones. These imaginary lines were then related to the skeleton. We found that, in practice, three lines sufficed for this division, and they could be related to well known anatomical landmarks. They are:

the first in the upper region of the shoulder girdle;
the second in the region of the lower costal margin, the waistline;
the third at the level of the pelvic floor.

These three transverse zones are shown in diagram 1 (page 21). With the help of this *vertical-horizontal framework,* the organs of the body are found lying in one of its three main compartments:

● The structures of the *head and neck* lie above the horizontal line drawn along the shoulder girdle.

● The *thorax and upper abdomen* with their organs lie within the region bounded by the horizontal lines of the shoulder girdle superiorly, and the waistline inferiorly.

● The organs of the *abdomen and pelvis* lie within the region bounded by the horizontal lines of the waistline above and the pelvic floor below.

The Zone Grid on the Feet

For the purposes of reflex zone massage to the feet, the following relationships between the body zones and the reflex zones on the feet are found.

(a) *The vertical body zones* divide the feet from heel to toe into ten fields, which correspond to the ten zones of the body, in which are incorporated all the organs of the head and trunk.

Generally, the reflex zone to an organ occupies the same vertical body zone in the feet as that organ occupies in the body, and should be looked for here.

Examples: The right shoulder girdle — vertical zones 4 and 5 on the right side of the body — finds its corresponding reflex zone in the feet in the same fourth and fifth vertical body zones around the joint of the small toe of the right foot. (See diagram 2: The bones of the feet — pages 24 and 25).

The left kidney — vertical zones 2 and 3 on the left — has its reflex zone in the vertical body zones 2 and 3 of the left foot, in the region of the proximal end of the second and third metatarsal bones.

The spine — vertical body zone 1 on the right and left of the body — is reflected in body zones 1 of the feet, that is to say along the longitudinal arch of both soles.

In the same way, all the organs of the body find their reflex zones on the feet in the corresponding vertical body zone.

(b) *The three transverse zones* are employed in the same fashion to divide the feet. The transverse zones represent not only the division of the body into three parts, but also a similar division of the feet. These are easily recognized because of their correlation to anatomical features, and are as follows:

Reflex zones to the structures of the *head and neck* are found in the area of the phalanges of *all the toes*. The first transverse line on the foot passes through the joints formed by the articulation of all the metatarsal bones and the phalanges of the toes, and corresponds to the transverse line drawn at the level of the shoulder girdle.

Reflex zones to the organs and structures of the *thorax and upper abdomen* are found in the anatomical region of the five *metatarsal bones* of either foot, and are bounded by Lisfranc's joint line, along which partial amputation of the foot is customarily performed. This second transverse line corresponds to the transverse division of the body at the waistline.

Reflex zones to the organs and structures of the *abdomen and pelvis* are found over the area of the tarsal bones, up to and including the inner and outer malleoli. This third transverse line corresponds to that of the body at the level of the pelvic floor and hip joint.

By so dividing the feet into imaginary vertical and transverse zones one constructs a grid into which each zone fits as chips of stone into a mosaic.

The lines which from the vertical zones of the body divide the body equally and bilaterally as they run from head to foot, and they do not cross over in the neck.

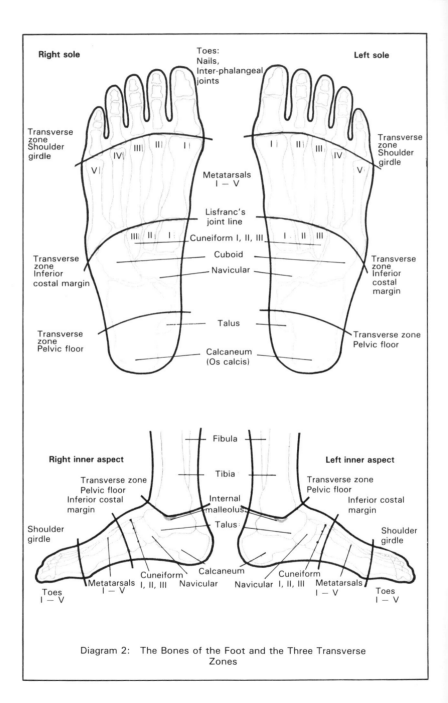

Right sole

Toes:
Nails,
Inter-phalangeal
joints

Left sole

Transverse
zone
Shoulder
girdle

IIII III II I
VI
IV

I II III
IV
V

Transverse
zone
Shoulder
girdle

Metatarsals
I – V

Lisfranc's
joint line

IIII II I Cuneiform I, II, III I II III

Cuboid

Navicular

Transverse
zone
Inferior
costal margin

Transverse
zone
Inferior
costal
margin

Talus

Transverse
zone
Pelvic floor

Transverse zone
Pelvic floor

Calcaneum
(Os calcis)

Fibula

Right inner aspect

Tibia

Left inner aspect

Transverse zone
Pelvic floor
Inferior costal
margin

Internal
malleolus

Transverse zone
Pelvic floor
Inferior costal
margin

Talus

Shoulder
girdle

Shoulder
girdle

Cuneiform
I, II, III

Calcaneum
Navicular

Cuneiform
Navicular I, II, III

Metatarsals
I – V

Toes
I – V

Metatarsals
I – V

Toes
I – V

Diagram 2:   The Bones of the Foot and the Three Transverse
Zones

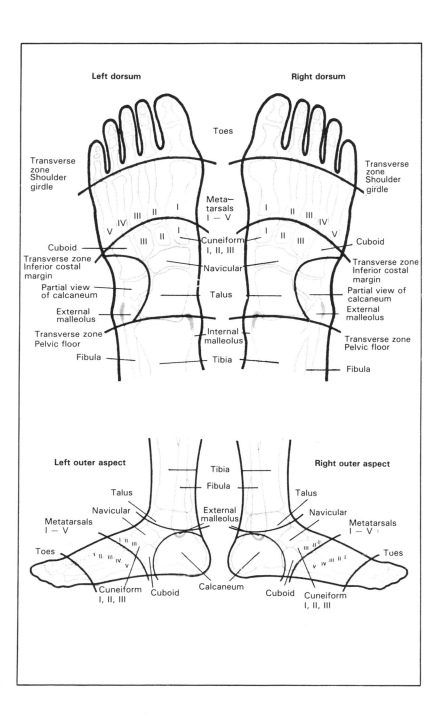

Left dorsum

Right dorsum

Toes

Transverse
zone
Shoulder
girdle

Transverse
zone
Shoulder
girdle

Meta-
tarsals
I – V

I

III II I

II III IV

V IV I

I

III II

II III

V

Cuboid

Cuneiform
I, II, III

Cuboid

Transverse zone
Inferior costal
margin

Transverse zone
Inferior costal
margin

Navicular

Partial view
of calcaneum

Partial view of
calcaneum

Talus

External
malleolus

External
malleolus

Transverse zone
Pelvic floor

Internal
malleolus

Transverse zone
Pelvic floor

Fibula

Tibia

Fibula

Left outer aspect

Right outer aspect

Tibia

Fibula

Talus

Talus

Navicular

External
malleolus

Navicular

Metatarsals
I – V

Metatarsals
I – V

Toes

I II III

I II III IV V

III II I

V IV III II I

Tues

Cuneiform
I, II, III

Cuboid

Calcaneum

Cuboid

Cuneiform
I, II, III

3.
THE CONCEPT OF REFLEX ZONES

The term 'reflex zone' has long been used in manual therapies, most frequently in connection with neurological reflexes. '*Connective tissue massage*' has also been described as 'work in the reflectory zones of the connective tissue'.[1,2]

At the end of the last century, Head and Mackenzie had already described such reflectory relationships between the periphery of the body and its internal organs.

According to a leading medical dictionary *Pschyrembel*,[3] the word 'reflex' in the strict medical sense means an involuntary muscle contraction due to an external stimulus and relayed by a central organ such as the spinal cord (B. Rückenmark).

In the context of reflex zones to the feet, the work 'reflex' is not used in this sense, but in its twin meanings:

(i)   As reflecting the entire organism (head, neck and trunk) on a small screen (the feet), rather like a reflex camera.

(ii)   In particular, in characteristic sections of the feet, which have been shown empirically to have a direct energy relationship with the internal organs.

This has nothing to do with Head and Mackenzie, or connective tissue massage, or the energy network of acupuncture. These systems have their own network and rules which regulate their performance. That we know as much as we do today, yet still do not understand that energy system which is presumably derived from the metabolic pathways which are essential to life, is already a familiar fact.

In order not to confuse the reader by charting the overlapping points of the different systems on the feet, only the outline of the feet with its skeletal structure has been shown in the diagrams, without introducing the muscles, tendons, vessels and meridians. The reflex zones have thus been represented in isolation and separated from their natural place in the living tissues which normally envelop them, but this does make the method easier to learn.

In practice, the therapist is going to work on the reflexes to the nerve roots emerging from the lumbar and sacral segments of the spine (on the feet) without performing connective tissue massage; and will encounter acupuncture points without doing acupuncture. Similarly the periosteum of the bone will be probed without doing periosteal massage, and lymphatic reservoirs will be massaged without your actually practising lymphatic drainage.

The concept of treatment through working on the zones of the feet (reflex zone therapy) arose when the concept of the body zones (zone therapy) was integrated by Dr W. Fitzgerald who developed the one from the other.

4.
REVIEW OF THE REFLEX ZONES OF THE FEET

It is frequently assumed that only the soles of the feet are important in reflex zone massage, as they were more usually portrayed in the early pictures and diagrams. In fact the *whole* foot, plantar and dorsal surfaces up to and including the inner and outer malleoli should be included in a complete treatment.

From the *soles* of the feet one may become aware of many things, particularly if one is a beginner, and they provide an outlook from which a total picture may be derived, as well as making it easier to think in a three dimensional way.

The feet must be considered as a *unity*, and not as two separate entities. The entire portrait of the body can be seen true to scale in the feet, bearing in mind that only the head, neck and trunk are being mirrored in the feet, the extremities being absent. An aid to this presentation is given in the following diagram:

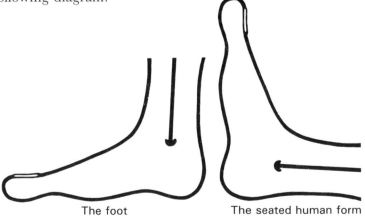

The foot   The seated human form

Diagram 3

As a general rule, it may be stated that every organ has a corresponding reflex zone in the feet, lying in the same zone in the feet as in the body. *Overlapping* of the reflex zones accords with the overlapping of the organs which occurs anatomically. Thus you find:

The organs of the right half of the body in the right foot, and the organs of the left side of the body in the left foot;

Organs which are paired in the body are also found in their corresponding zones on the left and right foot;

Single organs are found once only, in either left or right foot, and conform to their anatomical position;

Organs which lie in the centre of the body are found in both feet on their medial aspects.

The actual reflex zones terminate at the level of the ankle joint. Experience has shown, however, that treating areas which lie within a hand's breadth above the ankle joint can have great therapeutic value. Here lie indirect reflex zones affecting the muscles and nerves of the *lower extremities,* and those having some bearing on the origin of muscles and on nerves *within* the pelvis. They are described as '*indirect zones*'.

The *indirect reflex zones* to the *upper extremities* as far as the shoulder lie along the lateral border of the fifth metatarsal bone on either foot, where they may be palpated. The muscles and nerve supply of the arms are enclosed here.

Note: In general the reflex zones to the *organs* can be readily palpated on the *plantar* aspect of the foot, whilst those to *bones, muscles* and *nerves* lie on the *dorsal* aspect.

Because of the closely woven fabric of the connective tissue on the plantar heel, it is usually left out of treatment, except in children and those with tender feet. There is no therapeutic disadvantage in this, for these zones, which are the reflex zones to the pelvic organs, can be as well treated on the rim or either side of the heel as far as the ankle joint. From this approach a less vigorous massage is necessary for proper treatment.

5.

POSITIONING THE PATIENT

The correct positioning the the patient is necessary before giving reflex zone massage to the feet. This will also considerably enhance the effects of your treatment. The following surroundings and equipment are advisable:

A well ventilated, clean and warm room.

Adequate space for patient and therapist.

A wide, well upholstered couch or massage table.

Any disturbing background noise should be eliminated.

Cushions for head, neck and knees should be used as necessary.

A light blanket (preferably not of synthetic fabric) with which to cover the patient, as

(a)   some loss of body heat accompanies each massage;

(b)   the patient finds it easier to relax in an atmosphere of personal attention; and

(c)   the patient will be less shy of allowing the legs to relax and fall into the necessary outwardly rotated position.

When the patient is lying down comfortably, any constricting clothing should be personally loosened (belt, brassiere, corset, collar, tie, trousers) so that he or she may breathe easily and freely. The patient should remove his or her watch.

The patient should lie in a supine position with the head slightly raised. This also enables the therapist to constantly observe the facial expression and any spontaneous reaction, whether of pain or relaxation, and consequently regulate the massage appropriately. From this position the patient may also view the therapist at work. This is of the greatest importance at the start of treatment in order to build up a relationship of trust.

6.
THE GRIP-SEQUENCE

People have become accustomed nowadays to the idea that a 'technique' is necessary to the performance of any therapy, and we say breathing technique, movement technique, massage technique, etc. The use of this word can be restrictive, and for our purpose is better avoided, for 'technique' can imply solely the mechanical and the material, and implicit in its use is a limitation to these two aspects.

Human beings inhabit three dimensions, even in their locomotion. Because of the existence of joints, movements are fluid and curved when the original upright posture is maintained, and not stiff and angular. Yet there is, unfortunately, the possibility of movements being performed in a two dimensional and restricted manner. The fluidity of movement is then lost, muscles become overstretched and malaligned, and the flowing dynamic co-ordination of each part becomes obstructed. This can be true of small as well as large joints.

Therefore, to start with, the hands of the therapist must be rightly positioned, whether lying in the quiet resting state or in the working position. The feet are held always in a natural, loose and relaxed position, without overstretching the muscles or rigidly fixing the joints.

The thumb adopts a special position facing the fingers. Because of its great flexibility, the therapist is able to encircle the foot of the patient, and literally to 'take it into his hands'. When working on the sole with the thumb, the fingers support the dorsum of the foot and vice versa. Because of its greater strength, and because it has a greater radius of movement from its base joint than do the fingers, the thumb is preferred during treatment, and especially so when one is a beginner.

There are two phases in the grip sequence, the active and the passive phase. The impulse for the active phase begins in the palm of the hand, which may be compared to an energy sea which feeds and directs each finger, rather than in the periphery of the individual working digit. As the active phase is initiated the thumb moves from its relaxed passive position in a curved, bowing movement into the tissue depths, taking on strength and intensity and growing in flexion, maintaining throughout a wide arc at its base joint. From this position of maximum activity the thumb is allowed to return passively from the tissue depths to its original position on the skin surface and resume the slack resting position of the passive stage.

Continually alternating these active and passive phases, the thumb proceeds, millimetre by millimetre, across the surface of the skin and the underlying reflex zones, giving rise to an undulating rhythm and a flowing energy distribution in the painful tissues of the feet.

The thumb should always move forward, and never lose contact with the surface of the skin during the treatment sequence. If the therapist attempts to move the thumb backwards, i.e. towards his own body rather than away from it, the smooth flowing movement becomes disjointed and is impeded. Whether a reflex zone is treated from left to right or from heel to toe is of secondary importance; the approach is dictated by the state of tissue tonus.

When the thumb of the therapist is kinked to a right angle the movement is incorrect, as the forward flowing movement becomes rigid and angular, and the thumb-nails will then come into contact with the skin surface, giving rise to unnecessary pain. Furthermore, this leads to a mechanical pressure which tires the therapist more rapidly and does not properly allow the patient's tissue time for regeneration, thereby exhausting the patient.

Even when the thumb-nail does not make contact with the tissues of the feet, the sharp, prickling pain of disturbed reflex zones will frequently give rise to a mistaken belief in the patient's mind that it is the therapist's nails which are the cause, for he is unable to distinguish between the injury from the outside and the sensation of pain in his own tissues. When this happens, it is essential that the patient can rely on the explanation of the therapist, and that he has a sense of being correctly treated.

In skilled and experienced hands the grip-sequence has the capacity for being transformed. It is because of this change from a slow progress across the individual reflex zones of the feet into a vital therapy of the disordered systems of the body that Reflex Zone Therapy derives its validity. This is so even when the patient suffers severe impairment of the tissues owing to disease or injury in more than one system, and treatment must be carefully integrated. There are similar development parallels with other methods in which treatment must be graduated and modified according to circumstances. Even Vicar Kneipp,[6] (a famous pastor in Germany who invented a specific form of cold water therapy) recounted that 'I had to put aside my earlier drastic applications . . . and I was converted from great mildness to even greater mildness in my cures.'

The neutral grip-sequence can be enhanced in two ways by varying:

1. Working *rhythm* and *tempo*;
2. *Intensity*, which depends on the amount of energy expended.

This allows the practitioner to choose between any one of four variations:

(a) Slow and deliberate
(b) Swift and uninterrupted   } variations in rhythm
(c) Gentle and encroaching
(d) Strong and stimulating   } variations in intensity

It should not be thought that the hand has only muscular strength to deliver, but should be remembered that it has the resource to work effectively with dexterity and a delicate strength which is not bound to visible muscular power.

There is no fixed rule for determining what should be the intensity and what the expenditure of energy in any given treatment. No two people react in the same way, and one person will react differently from the same stimulus as his internal and external circumstances alter. In general, one works up to the level of the individual patient's pain threshold, and only then, when the pain diminishes and is overcome, can tissue turgor begin to return to normal. (See section dealing with reactions.)

Neither can there be any rigid dictates as to the duration of each grip-sequence, that is, the length of time that pressure is exerted during the active phase. In earlier times painful stimuli of some minutes duration were advocated; today a second-long impulse frequently suffices to bring about a regenerative effect. These second-long impulses are repeated several times during a reflex zone massage in order to bring the tissues into a healthier state of tonus.

If the patient is in great pain, much debilitated or overwrought, even careful pressure on a reflex zone may then breach the pain threshold. This is more likely to happen when the patient is in a weakened nervous state (whether this is temporary or of long standing is beside the point), or when an organ is in the acute reactive phase. Pay very careful attention here, and use just that degree of pressure which calms and restores the patient. Frequently and gently stretch and stroke the feet and legs.

Once the fingers have become more receptive they are also able to execute fine vibratory and stretching movements in appropriate areas of the feet. The reactions caused by these specific grips are due to the swinging elasticity and rhythmical intrusion into the tissues of the finger-tips.

The Sedation Grip

When treating patients with acute pain (colic, acute earache, neuralgia, haemorrhoids, injuries, toothache, etc.), the movement is so adapted that it alleviates pain and calms the patient. This is accomplished by using a firm hold, which is sustained for 2-3 minutes, when fingers and thumbs maintain an even pressure in the painful tissues. It often happens that the pain in an organ subsides or disappears within a short time, that is as soon as the spasm is relieved in the reflex zone.

This sedation grip may be used as a form of 'first aid', and the fact that you may need to use it during a treatment does not exclude the possibility of your continuing to treat other organs and systems in order to seek out the underlying cause of the patient's condition (working, of course, always within the limits of the patient's tolerance).

7.

TREATMENT PROCEDURE

The feet should lie in such a position that they are within easy reach of the relaxed and erectly seated practitioner. The distance between the feet of the patient and the practitioner is dictated by the length of the loosely flexed arms. The patient's feet rest on the massage table, and must not be supported on the knees or thighs of the therapist. The manner of working must be so relaxed and flexible that if, at any time during the treatment, the patient wishes to withdraw his feet he may do so, and does not feel that he must helplessly endure the pain. He is likely, otherwise, to become anxious, cramped, tense or angry.

True pain will disturb the patient less when he is able to breathe easily and freely, and when he opens himself up as much as possible to the therapy. This also enables him to follow the massage procedure with attention and interest, and not to believe that his attention should be diverted through chatter or by misdirected concentration or relaxation exercises. He can, if he wishes, be wholly attentive to events at the site of therapy as they are being experienced in his feet.

The therapist establishes contact by taking the feet in her hands, and at the same time making a few gentle *stroking* movements. From this is gained the *first impression* of the following factors:

temperature;

dynamics of the feet (bony structure);

tissue turgor;

condition of the skin.

During the massage *both* hands should always be on the foot. Whilst one hand works, the other supports and maintains contact. With much experience and practice the grip sequence can be used bimanually and the fingers will be used in massage.

The practical activity and training of the instruction courses should be continually remembered; the experience of palpation cannot be theoretically transmitted.

In order to assess the *correct pressure* to discover what findings palpation may yield, note the spontaneous reactions of the patient to the *first* impulse of pressure. If the foot is jerked backwards or an involuntary expression of pain escapes, the intensity of your massage must be immediately reduced. If the patient is calm and still, or has the sensation of being lightly tickled, the individual pain threshold has not been reached.

When the appropriate intensity of your massage grip sequence has been found, one which the patient finds bearable, this measure is more or less kept to for the duration of the treatment, for it corresponds to the immediate condition of the entire person before you.

Note: People react differently to the same therapeutic stimulus, according to their own personal disease background. The same person will respond differently to the same therapy from time to time because of any of a number of changes in the inner and outer environment, such as:

change of climate;

active or passive phase of personal biorhythms:

change of diet;

emotional state;

early, and as yet unremarked, stages of many illnesses;

commencement of the reaction stage and healing crisis.

An evenly sustained pressure applied to different areas of the feet will elicit startling variations in sensation, and allow one to compare the differences between healthy tissues and disturbed reflex zones.

Treatment is most effective when the second long pressure impulse is repeated at frequent intervals, and not continuously, to the same area during a reflex zone massage. With each *repetition* the area will be less painful, which will be due in part to the improvement in circulation which follows massage.

Treatment is complete when the intense local pain in the disturbed reflex zones decreases to a level which is bearable for the patient. This usually happens within 20 – 30 minutes, but there will always be exceptions, and one patient may require only 15 minutes and another up to 50 minutes before the tissue tonus begins to be restored to normal.

The first reflex zone massage to the feet usually needs approximately 40 – 50 minutes, during which time an objective picture of the general condition of the feet must be built up from the symptoms as they are presented.

Thorough palpation of all reflex zones during the first treatment is more readily accomplished if the therapist has a well defined *concept of the order* in which the reflex zones are being treated. In this way, her work is systematically composed and she is less likely to overlook or forget those zones which she has discovered to be abnormal on visual examination.

Treatment always includes *both feet.* The reflex zones of the left and right foot are alternately massaged, and there is not an aimless or haphazarded drift from one place to another over the feet, but the systems of the body are treated in the appropriate sequence.

I recommend the following sequence, the effectiveness of which has been proven in practice:

(i)   **The Reflex Zones of the Head** (Diagram 4)

These display one marked peculiarity. Whilst they are distributed over all ten toes, the reflex zones of the head are further replicated in miniature on both large toes. For this reason, treatment of the reflex zones of the head begins on the two big toes.

Rotation of the big toe around the metatarso-phalangeal joint is the reflex equivalent of rotating the atlas on the axis, (that is the head on the neck). Any minute deposits which are present may make themselves heard or felt during such rotation through pain, crackling, friction, or by limitation of movement, and they all point to a corresponding disorder in the region of the head and/or neck.

The pad of the big toe represents the posterior aspect of the head, whilst its dorsal surface bears the reflex zones which

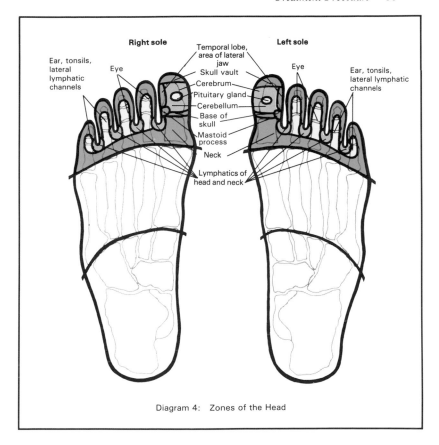

Diagram 4:   Zones of the Head

represent the face. The transverse crease which marks the proximal boundary of the pad of the big toe is the reflex zone which accords with the base of the skull.

The areas corresponding to the nose, mouth and throat occupy a relatively large area on the dorsum of the big toe, the surrounding tissues represent the bones and musculature of the face.

When these areas have been treated on the big toes, the reflex zones to these same structures are treated on the individual toes, where they are found in larger scale. Those reflex zones which correspond to the eyes and ears are best approached from the soles, whilst the sinuses and teeth may be treated from both plantar and dorsal aspects.

The reflex zones to the teeth are also exactly distributed over

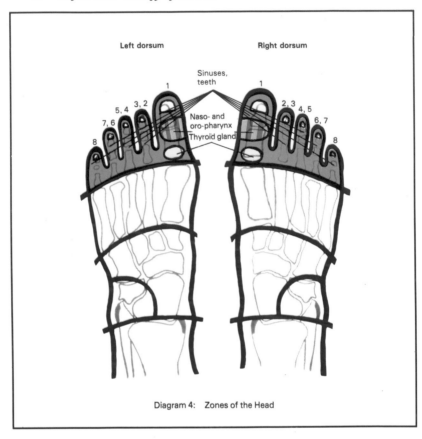

Left dorsum

Right dorsum

Sinuses,
teeth

1

1

5, 4 3, 2

2, 3 4, 5

7, 6

Naso- and
oro-pharynx

6, 7

8

Thyroid gland

8

Diagram 4:   Zones of the Head

the ten zones spanning the toes, and are arranged as follows:

Incisors	(1) —	Body zone 1 — Big toe
Incisors and canine teeth	(2, 3) —	Body zone 2 — Second toe
Premolars	(4, 5) —	Body zone 3 — Third toe
Molars	(6, 7) —	Body zone 4 — Fourth toe
Wisdom teeth	(8) —	Body zone 5 — Fifth toe

Important: During treatment, both medial and lateral sides of the toes are naturally included, even though they are not shown on the diagrams.

The tissue forming the webs of the toes reflects the upper lymphatic system, and a good blood supply to these areas is achieved by taking them in a pincer grasp and drawing firmly towards you, at the same time gently flexing the ball of the foot. (This movement is similar to that used when milking!) In the interests of hygiene, and in order not to spread infection, these areas are not treated in people with athlete's foot or other fungal infections until the infection has been cured.

(ii) **Reflex Zones to the Musculo-skeletal System** (Diagram 5)

(a) Spinal column
The reflex zones to the spinal column are situated along the longitudinal arches of the medial aspect of both feet.

- Those of the *cervical spine* are found along the entire length of the proximal phalanx of each big toe, beginning just a little distally to the interphalangeal joint which is the reflex zone to the base of the skull.

- Those of the *thoracic (or dorsal) spine* are found along the medial aspect of the first metatarsal bone of either foot.

- Those of the *lumbar spine* are found along the medial aspect of the first cuneiform bone and the distal half of the scaphoid bone.

- Those of the *sacrum* from the proximal part of the scaphoid bone and along part of the talus on their medial aspects.

- Those of the *coccyx* along the distal third of the calcaneum.

These reflex zones are not massaged by applying pressure to the periosteum or along the ridge of the bone but in the muscles which clothe them, slightly towards the sole. There are, however, certain reflex zones to the nervous system which lie along the periosteum of the bone.
Note: Reflex zone massage before treatment by a chiropractor has proven to be useful. Intense muscular spasm treated by reflex zone massage preparatory to manipulation of the vertebrae ensures that the procedure is less painful to the patient and requires less energetic manipulation. From time to time muscles and tendons which have been relaxed in this way permit a vertebra to slip back into position (usually a cervical vertebra)

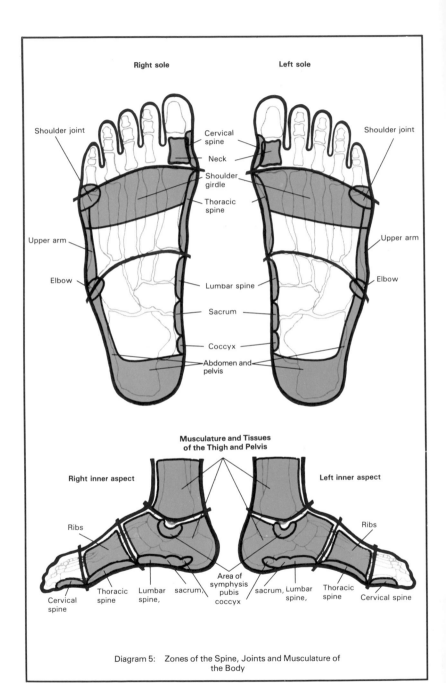

Diagram 5:   Zones of the Spine, Joints and Musculature of
the Body

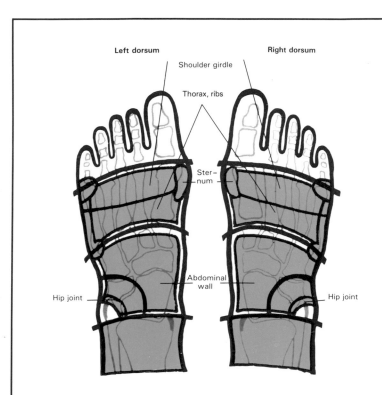

Left dorsum   **Right dorsum**

Shoulder girdle

Thorax, ribs

Ster-
num

Abdominal
wall

Hip joint   Hip joint

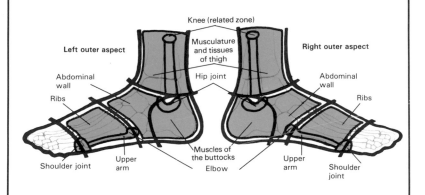

Knee (related zone)

Musculature
and tissues
of thigh

Left outer aspect   Hip joint   **Right outer aspect**

Abdominal   Abdominal
wall   wall

Ribs   Ribs

Shoulder joint   Upper   Muscles of   Upper   Shoulder
                   arm   the buttocks   arm   joint
                            Elbow

during reflex zone massage to the feet, and may be heard and felt by the patient returning to its normal position.

The joint formed by the phalanx of the big toe and the first metatarsal bone (i.e. the reflex zone to the lower cervical and upper thoracic spine) requires careful observation. This joint often shows pathological changes in the form of a *hallux valgus* (lateral flexion of the big toe). Due to the altered alignment of the bones in this area, the reflex zones to the neck are affected. Observation of hundreds of patients has shown that when a *hallux valgus* is present, there is nearly always concommitant tension of the neck and shoulder muscles, and/or dysfunction of the thyroid gland.

The physical distortion of bone and muscle structure, (and all its effects in the skeletal, postural and supporting systems) forms a pathological picture which has been supplemented by the empirical experience of reflex zone massage.

(b)   Reflex zones of the neck and shoulder girdle

These are found spanning the transverse arches formed by the distal halves of the metatarsal bones on both plantar and dorsal aspects. When the reflex zone to the right shoulder is worked on from the plantar aspect, the reflex zones to the liver and gall-bladder are indirectly treated at the same time; and with the left shoulder girdle the reflex zone to the heart will be simultaneously indirectly treated, (because of their related segmental innervation).

The reflex zone to the *shoulder girdle* on the *dorsum* of the feet has long been known. It overlies the distal half of all five metatarsal bones (as described above), and this area should be inlcluded in all treatment to the shoulder girdle, corresponding as it does to the ventral surface of the thorax. It is actually more correctly described as the *indirect* reflex zone to the shoulder girdle, but experience has shown that once tension in the interstices between the metatarsal bones on the dorsum of the feet has been alleviated, the musculature and nerve tracts of the shoulder girdle can be more competently treated.

Note: A special relationship has been found to be present in the shoulder girdle between the physical and the mental. Muscular rigidity and decreased flexibility of the transverse arches betoken not only a physical disorder, but are also an indication of the psychical or stress burden that people have to 'carry on their shoulders'.

Treatment Procedure   45

The reflex zone which corresponds to the *shoulder joint* is easily recognized in the feet, mirrored in the articulation of each small toe with the fifth metatarsal bone.

Although only the head, neck and trunk are reflected in their three dimensions in the shape, form and structure of the feet, the elbow and knee joints can be treated through an *indirect* reflex zone which is located on the feet. In this way the lateral borders of the fifth metatarsal bones are, on the one hand, the reflex zone to the lateral aspect of the thorax, and on the other hand the indirect reflex zone to the *upper arm* as far as the *elbow* joint, which lies at the base of the fifth metatarsal bone.

The reflex zone to the *sternum* is situated on the distal dorsal surface of the first metatarsal bone. There is a relationship between this zone and those of the heart, organs of respiration, lymphatic system and the alignment of the spinal column.

The *ribs* and musculature of the thorax extend over the whole area formed by the metatarsal bones on plantar and dorsal aspects of both feet.

As the reflex zones to the head are found in both small and larger scale on the ten toes, this rule is found to be true for the reflex zones to the *neck* as well. Thus the reflex zone to the neck is found in its small scale just below the pad of the large toe ventrally, and fans out in its larger scale on the ten body zones on the lower part of each toe at its base joint.

(c) The pelvic girdle
The reflex zones to the pelvic girdle extend over the area of the tarsal bones and heel, up to and including the inner and outer malleoli. The region from cuboid bone to outer malleolus bears the reflex zones to the lateral bones and musculature of the *pelvis*. The area directly inferior to the inner malleoli corresponds to the *symphysis pubis,* the area overlying the articulating surfaces of the fibula, talus and tibia is the reflex zone to the *hip joint* on either foot.

As the indirect zone to the elbow could be traced from the shoulder joint, the *indirect* zone to the *knee* can be found located on the fibula, at a point directly superior to the outer malleolus; and the indirect zone to the thigh between these two points, as well as posteriorly to the fibula.

A reflex zone to the knee has been known for decades, lying on the lateral rim of the heel, directly inferior to the outer malleolus. Logically, this should be a reflex zone to the pelvic region according to the anatomical correspondence of this area with the pelvis. However, due to the fact that this is also a reflex zone to the nerves which supply the leg, the knee can be treated here through its indirect reflex zone.

Many years of observation have shown that in acute conditions the reflex zone on the fibula reacts sensitively, whilst in chronic disease processes the reflex zone on the rim of the lateral heel is extremely painful as well.

(iii) Reflex Zones to the Urinary System (Diagram 6)

In treating the reflex zones of the urinary system, either the functional arrangement of the organs may be followed, i.e. by proceeding from kidney to ureter then bladder; or, since the bladder is not just a toneless hollow receptacle for urine, but also one of the organs of excretion in that it retains and voids urine, by working from bladder to ureter to kidney.

The anatomical background to the reflex zones of the *kidneys* is the base of both the second and third metatarsal bones on the soles of the feet. The tendon of the *hallucis longus* muscle serves as an orientation line for the reflex zone to the *ureter*. Since the *bladder* is situated in the centre of the pelvis, its reflex zone is found lying below the inner malleolus on both feet.

Note: The tendon to the *hallucis longus* muscle is easily visible when the big toe is flexed dorsally, and runs from underneath the pad of the big toe as far as the heel. The tendon is not worked on whilst it is thus extended, but along its medial corner when the toes have been returned to their normal position.

The nervous pathways to the lumbar spine and the bladder are so well known that it will be realized, when treating the reflex zone to the bladder, that the lumbar spine will be treated at the same time, lying as it does directly behind the bladder.

(iv) Reflex Zones to the Organs of Digestion (Diagram 7)

The digestive tract begins at the *mouth,* whose reflex zone lies on the dorsal aspect of the big toe. From here the reflex zone to the *oesophagus* tracks proximally (on both plantar and dorsal aspects), having as its boundary the metatarso-phalangeal joint. The *stomach* is best treated towards the base of the first metatarsal

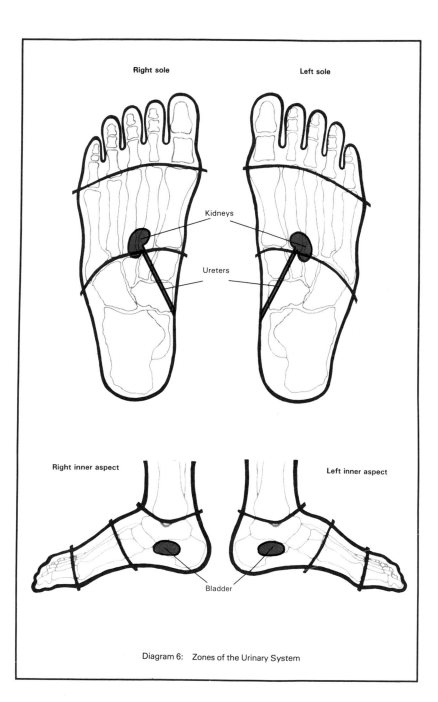

Right sole

Left sole

Kidneys

Ureters

Right inner aspect

Left inner aspect

Bladder

Diagram 6: Zones of the Urinary System

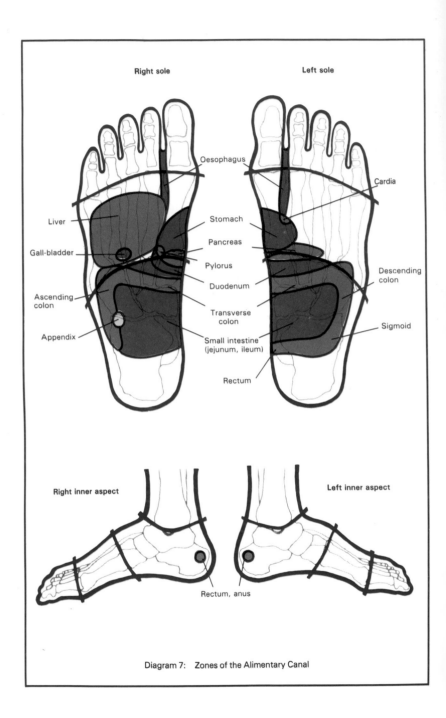

Right sole

Left sole

Oesophagus

Cardia

Liver

Stomach

Gall-bladder

Pancreas

Pylorus

Duodenum

Descending colon

Ascending colon

Transverse colon

Appendix

Small intestine (jejunum, ileum)

Sigmoid

Rectum

Right inner aspect

Left inner aspect

Rectum, anus

Diagram 7: Zones of the Alimentary Canal

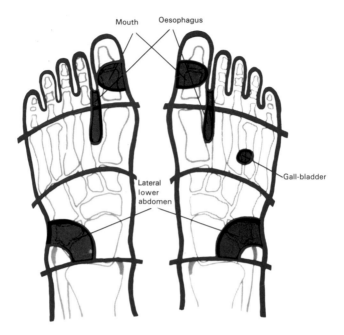

Left dorsum

Right dorsum

Mouth

Oesophagus

Gall-bladder

Lateral
lower
abdomen

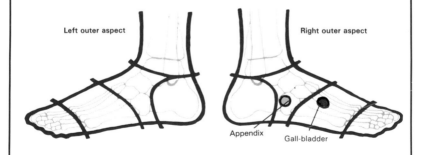

Left outer aspect

Right outer aspect

Appendix

Gall-bladder

bone on both right and left feet. The *cardia* on the left foot and the *pylorus* on the right may easily be differentiated.

The three segments of the *small intestine* are illustrated in the diagram. They are not so readily distinguished in practice as in an abstract drawing; as their form, length and size alter according to their content and muscular tone. Here again a discrepancy between theoretical representation and individual feet cannot be avoided. There are, however, two reliable *fixed points* which can be located, and which serve to orient the therapist. One is the *pylorus* (where the stomach ends and the small intestine begins), and the other the *ileo-caecal valve*, (which is the transition point from small to large intestine). Between these two points the coils of the small intestine are found spread out over the left and right soles.

Note: The zones of the small intestine are often easily recognized on visual observation of the soles when a fleshiness is noticed over the first, second and third cuneiform bones. (See diagram 2: Bones of the feet). In West Germany Dr H. Mozer[7] has frequently repositioned these bones because of some fault in their alignment. We have observed a number of patients in whom digestive function has markedly improved following this intervention, due to the fact that correct alignment of these bones of the feet has had a favourable influence on the reflex zones to the digestive tract.

By laying a finger across the sole of the right foot, starting from the base of the fifth metatarsal bone and directing it diagonally towards the heel, one will find, even on one's own foot, at a distance of one finger joint, the reflex zone to the *appendix*. Directly above this, on the dorsum of the foot, is a further reflex zone to the appendix, and this is often easier to treat. If there is greatly heightened sensitivity in this area combined with the symptoms of an acute abdomen, the patient's doctor should be informed, in case appendicitis is developing.

The reflex zones to the *pancreas* are difficult to find on the feet. Since this organ cannot be easily palpated in the abdomen, neither can its reflex zone be easily differentiated from those of other organs which are related to it. Some of its functions are closely allied to those of the organs of the upper abdomen, and the pancreas is treated simultaneously with the reflex zones to the stomach, duodenum and liver. When treating a patient with diabetes mellitus, it is necessary to work in close co-operation with the doctor, since insulin doses may sometimes need to be altered during treatment. The patient should also be instructed to take particular care in noting the sugar content of his or her urine during treatment.

The reflex zones to the *large intestine* start on the lateral side of the right foot over the area of the tarsal bones. From here the *ascending colon* tracks toward the midline of the foot, and the *transverse colon* lies transversely across all ten body zones of both left and right feet, as far as the lateral border of the left foot. From here the reflex zones to the *descending colon* track heelward, leading into the reflex zones to the *sigmoid colon, rectum and anus*. This area is of particular importance, since it is often extremely painful, even when the patient does not have any known rectal pathology. It may be an indication of undiagnosed anal eczema, diarrhoea, prolapsed rectum, tumour or other pelvic disease.

Note: Experience has shown that where there is an existing disorder of the autonomic nervous system, there is an associated constriction of all the sphincters in the body, and particularly of the anal sphincter. This region (the reflex zone to the rectum and anus) should therefore be palpated in every patient where there is a suggestion of such dysfunction for verification, and if necessary, treatment.

The reflex zone to the *liver* is situated on the sole of the right foot, and includes the reflex zone to the *gall-bladder* at its proximal boundary. The reflex zone to the gall-bladder is also found directly above this on the *dorsum* of the foot, where it is easier to locate.

Note: We have observed that when a haematoma occurs on the feet following therapy, the organs which correspond to that reflex zone are overtaxed or diseased, as may also happen with the reflex zone to the gall-bladder. When a bruise or haematoma is present on the feet, gently include the area in your treatment in order to relieve the congestion and pain.

(v)   Reflex Zones to the Organs of Respiration (Diagram 8)

The reflex zones to the respiratory system begin, as do those of the digestive tract, in the area corresponding to the *nose* and *mouth* on the dorsum of the big toe. From here the reflex zones to the *trachea* and *bronchi* are found laterally, towards the mid-point of the first and second metatarsal bones on both plantar and dorsal surfaces. From here they fan out over the large expanses which form the *bronchial* and *lung parenchymal* reflex zones,

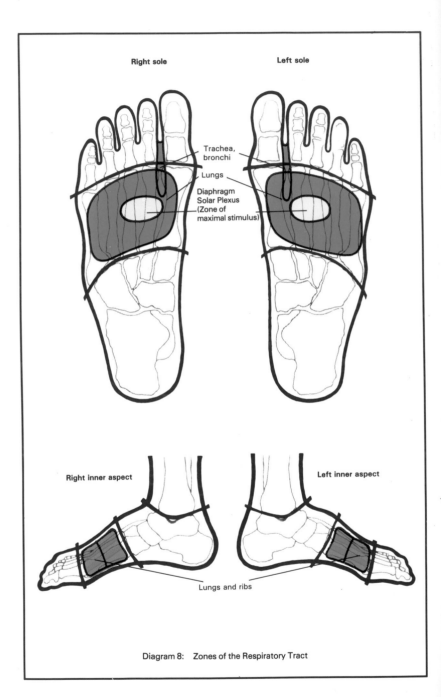

Right sole

Left sole

Trachea,
bronchi

Lungs

Diaphragm
Solar Plexus
(Zone of
maximal stimulus)

Right inner aspect

Left inner aspect

Lungs and ribs

Diagram 8:   Zones of the Respiratory Tract

Left dorsum

Right dorsum

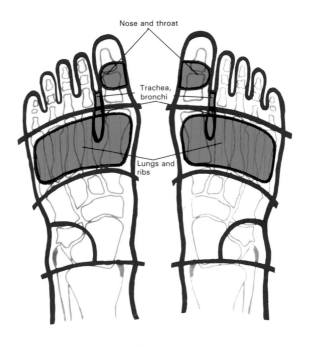

Nose and throat

Trachea, bronchi

Lungs and ribs

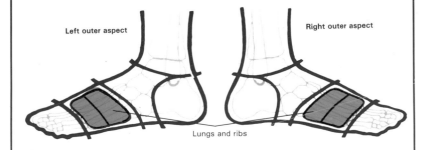

Left outer aspect

Right outer aspect

Lungs and ribs

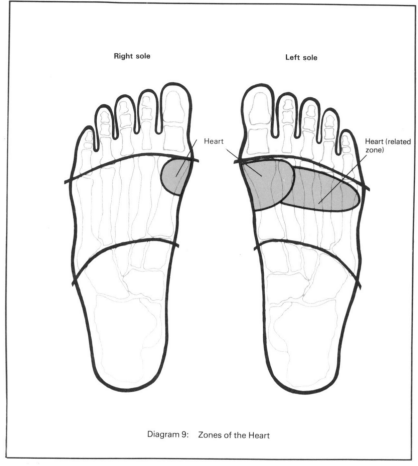

Diagram 9:   Zones of the Heart

encompassing the whole area of the foot formed by the metatarsal bones.

Although the *diaphragm* is a large domed muscle which defines the thorax inferiorly, there are two points where maximal stimulus to its reflex zones are affected. These lie directly beneath the transverse arches formed by the metatarsal bones in body zones 2 and 3. This reflex zone is also that of the *solar plexus*. Maximal stimulus to the solar plexus is likewise effected at this point, from where it fans out in a wave like fashion over the whole efferent network of the solar plexus.

Note: Those patients who are very weak and hardly able to bear the stimulus of a reflex zone massage as it would normally be carried out, respond positively to *repeated,* gentle pressure on the

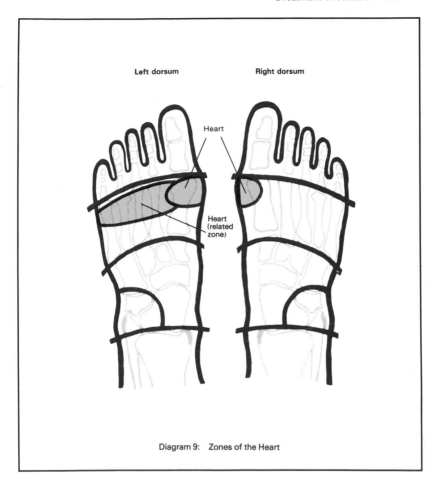

Left dorsum   Right dorsum

Heart

Heart
(related
zone)

Diagram 9:   Zones of the Heart

reflex zone to the diaphragm and solar plexus. This becomes even more effective when the *respiratory rhythm* is taken into account. The reflex zone to the diaphragm can be pressed gently yet firmly to the extent to which it is tolerable for the patient. On expiration the pressure is released. In this way the heightened sensitivity of the patient to pain is often overcome within a few minutes.

(vi) Reflex Zones to the Heart (Diagram 9)

The *heart* has both a reflex zone to the organ and a segmental indirect reflex zone. The reflex zone to the organ is bounded by the area which matches the sternum dorsally and the upper part of the thoracic spine on the plantar aspects of both feet. The *indirect reflex zone* lies laterally on the left sole. The indirect reflex zone to the heart and the reflex zone to the shoulder girdle are identical here, and also on the left dorsum, extending over the area which corresponds to the thorax, as far as the shoulder joint.

Experience has shown that better results are obtained from treating the indirect rather than the direct reflex zone to the heart. A parallel may be drawn here with many other forms of cutaneo-visceral and segmentally related forms of therapy.

The precept to follow when treating the reflex zones to the heart is: 'Depress hyperexcitability and stimulate flaccidity'. *Arndt-Schultz' basic biological precept,* 'Weak stimuli are beneficial, strong stimuli are detrimental, very strong stimuli are harmful' has particular relevance for patients with heart disease.

When treating a patient with heart disease the therapist can try to disassociate herself from thinking only of symptoms and consider casual relationships. In many cases, the organs of digestion, the dynamic equilibrium of the spinal column, or the endocrine glands share the origin of disorder with the heart, and are therefore important for this wider and more productive way of thinking.

(vii) The Reflex Zones to the Lymphatic System (Diagram 10)

The reflex zones to the lymphatics of the head and neck are found in the webs of the toes on both plantar and dorsal surfaces of the feet. Conspicuous amongst these is the reflex zone to the *tonsils,* situated on the lateral aspect of both big toes at their base. Today, this reflex zone is almost always sensitive in most people: nor does one have far to seek for the cause. The lymphatic system is the most vulnerable of the filtering systems of the human body. Personal and environmental pollution, dietary indiscretion, the abuse of drugs and chemicals all play their part in overtaxing this system, as do illnesses which have been suppressed by unwise drug administration.

Note: When treating the reflex zone to the tonsils it has often been noticed that they remain painful, even when the tonsils have been surgically removed. This seems at first paradoxical. There are two possible explanations:

1. When an organ is removed a scar remains, and this may subsequently give rise to a painful reflex zone. (The energy field in that area is disturbed.)

2. Even after surgical removal, an organ may exert a disturbing influence on the energy field which it formerly occupied. People who have lost a limb suffer phantom pains because of their altered bodily image, and it is this energy field which is being referred to here, although there is not the conscious awareness when an organ is removed. In the same way all other scars and focal infections may bring about a disturbing influence on the energy fields to which they are related.

An eminent doctor has said: 'After an operation the sick person is often the same sick person, but without the respective organ'. This is not to say that under circumstances which threaten life or where there are special indications, an operation should not be performed.

The reflex zones to the *axillary lymphatics* are found proximal to the shoulder joint on both plantar and dorsal surfaces. Those to the *lymphatics of the groin* lie in the dorsal transverse stretch between inner and outer malleoli, that is to say, between the reflex zones to the symphysis pubis and the hip joint.

The anatomical areas of the true pelvis and the upper thighs are richly endowed with lymphatic nodes and channels, and this is reflected on the medial and lateral aspects of the heel and in the area around the Achilles Tendon. Lymphatic congestion of the pelvis will be accurately mirrored over this part of the heel, which must be included in the treatment of the lymphatic system.

The reflex zone to the *spleen* is found at the bases of the third, fourth and fifth metatarsal bones on the plantar aspect of the left foot. According to our experience, pain is felt on pressure in the following cases:

> *acute and chronic infections and inflammatory processes:*
>
> *Blood dyscrasia (and any abnormality of blood components);*
>
> *in all forms of allergy,* and in any condition in which there is a predisposition to *myocardial infarction,* when it is often far more sensitive than would be expected.

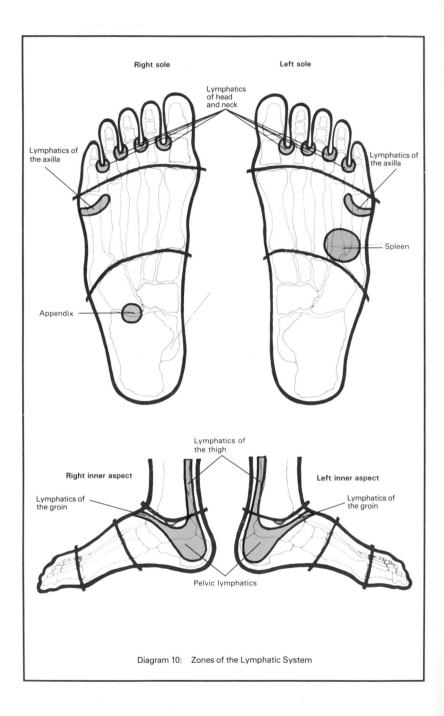

Right sole   Left sole

Lymphatics of head and neck

Lymphatics of the axilla

Lymphatics of the axilla

Spleen

Appendix

Lymphatics of the thigh

Right inner aspect   Left inner aspect

Lymphatics of the groin

Lymphatics of the groin

Pelvic lymphatics

Diagram 10: Zones of the Lymphatic System

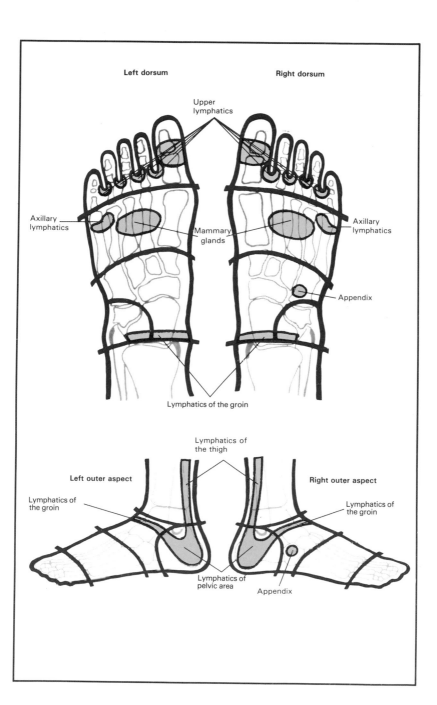

Left dorsum

Right dorsum

Upper
lymphatics

Axillary
lymphatics

Mammary
glands

Axillary
lymphatics

Appendix

Lymphatics of the groin

Lymphatics of
the thigh

Left outer aspect

Right outer aspect

Lymphatics of
the groin

Lymphatics of
the groin

Lymphatics of
pelvic area

Appendix

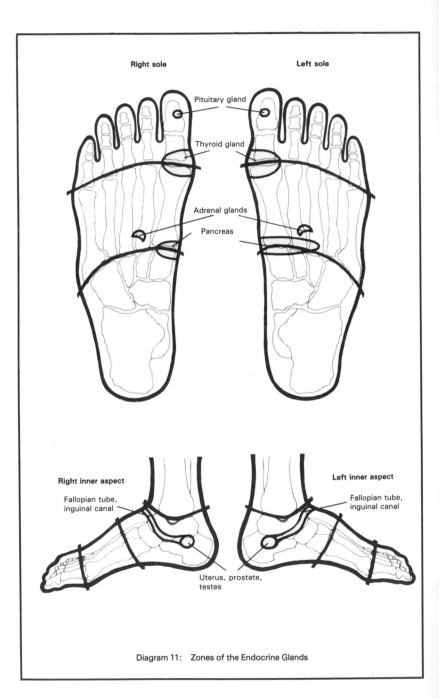

Diagram 11: Zones of the Endocrine Glands

Right sole

Left sole

Pituitary gland

Thyroid gland

Adrenal glands

Pancreas

Right inner aspect

Left inner aspect

Fallopian tube,
inguinal canal

Fallopian tube,
inguinal canal

Uterus, prostate,
testes

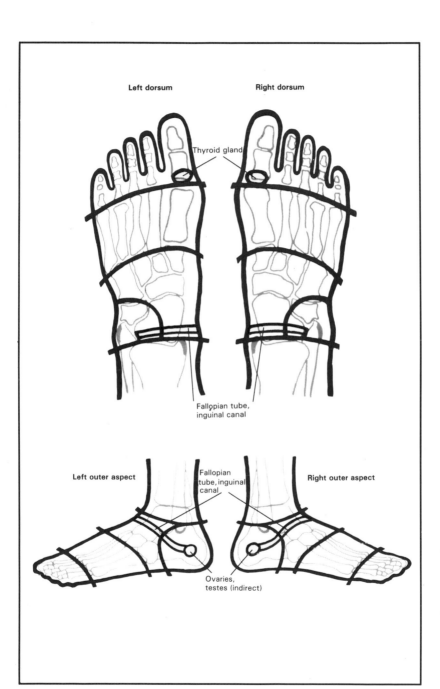

Left dorsum   Right dorsum

Thyroid gland

Fallopian tube,
inguinal canal

Left outer aspect

Fallopian
tube, inguinal
canal

Right outer aspect

Ovaries,
testes (indirect)

(viii) **Reflex Zones to the Endocrine System** (Diagram 11)

These zones are, as in the body, widely distributed over the feet. that of the *pituitary gland* lies on the pad of the big toe, at the centre of the concentrically arranged rings there (the papilla).

Note for blind therapists:
The location of these reflex zones is the highest point on the pad of the big toe (papilla), and they are readily distinguished on gentle palpation, even when they have been pushed to one side due to the weight of the body or too tight shoes.

The reflex zone to the *thyroid gland.* which coincides in part with those of the throat and larynx overlies the metatarso-phalangeal joints of both big toes on dorsal and plantar surfaces. In cases of disease, such as thyrotoxicosis, these areas should be treated with great care, since in these patients the autonomic nervous system reacts with hypersensitivity. The reflex zone to the *pancreas,* part endocrine gland and part organ of digestion, has already been described under the digestive tract.

It is scarcely possible to distinguish between the reflex zone to the *adrenal gland* and that of the kidney in either foot, since the adrenal is so closely related to the superior pole of the kidney. They are sensitive to touch, not only in cases of renal disease, but also in the whole spectrum of *rheumatic disease* and *allergies.*

The reflex zones to the *genitalia* are found both medially and laterally below the internal and external malleoli. On the medial aspect lie the reflex zones to the centrally located organs of the *uterus* and *vagina,* the *prostate* and *testes;* and on the lateral aspect those to the *ovaries.* As the testes descend through the inguinal canal, they may also be indirectly treated in this area.

Care for the health and well-being of women *during and after pregnancy* with reflex zone therapy to the feet is particularly rewarding, and beneficial to both mother and child. Normal pregnancy is not an illness, and after much experience no doubts remain about the benefit of such treatment. When the pregnancy is unstable or at risk, then any decision about treatment is taken by the doctor alone. Unhappily, women are not always well during their pregnancies. There may be visible congestion of the veins, lymphatics, or problems associated with altered stance and weightbearing which cause problems in the spinal column, heart, respiratory organs or digestive tract. These conditions respond extremely well to zone therapy. Delivery and the involution of organs in the puerperium are usually problem-free and spontaneously accomplished, and the period of lactation may be prolonged with appropriate reflex zone massage to the feet.

Note: It has been our experience that undescended testes (crypto-orchidism) in young boys may be successfully treated. It is a question of noting the causal reflex zones. (See Section 11 of the book: Case Histories.) Some parents do not take this youthful developmental disorder seriously enough.

The reflex zones to the *breasts* lie centrally on the dorsum of the feet, overlying the metatarsal bones. In cases of premenstrual tension (swelling and tenderness of the breasts before menstruation), reflex zone therapy usually relieves the symptoms until at least the next period. Tenderness of this area and related tenderness of the reflex zones to the genitalia and the axillary lymphatics demand further investigation of the underlying causes.

Summary
With the systematic working through of these eight systems of the body, which serve to provide one with a first *visual* and *palpable* set of *observations,* treatment is concluded.

At intervals during this sequence, depending on the character and response of the patient, include a few *gentle stroking* movements at times. When and where they should be inserted you will be able to judge from the reactions of the patient to the treatment as you proceed. These movements are particularly valuable in making your first contact with the feet, and in bringing the course of treatment to a quiet and calm termination.

At the end of treatment the feet should be *warm and pleasantly relaxed.* If this is not so, there are two possible reasons:

1. The dosage, intensity and duration of the treatment has not been graduated according to the tolerance of the individual patient.

2. The vitality and resistance of the patient are at such a low ebb that they are inadequate to produce enough body heat to warm the patient. Therefore it may happen that, despite a thorough and well-gauged treatment, the feet cannot be sufficiently warmed from within. In this type of case there is

a place for passive warming by the judicious use of footbaths, lightboxes, hot water bottles, etc., but only *after* the treatment.

A patient who is returning home with cold feet cannot expect any stabilization or regeneration of his or her condition. After a few treatments many patients become aware of the capacity of their own bodies to regulate and distribute body heat, and at the same time realize what progress is being made.

Along with stroking and warming movements, you may occasionally introduce into the treatment a sequence of movements which will relax and loosen the joints of the feet, particularly the toe joints, the metatarsal bones and the bones of the heels.

Note: Manipulation of the toes at their base joints requires special care. Adaptation of the inner pressure of the joint to atmospheric pressure is audible, and means that those joints are articulating at their normal tension. Practising this movement is useful for the following reasons:

1. Because these articulations of the toes with the metatarsal bones correspond to the upper border of the shoulder girdle, restoring them to normal function brings about a corresponding release in tension in the shoulder girdle.

2. The degree of anxiety which this movement provokes in the patient gives you an indication as to whether he is labile or in a state of equilibrium. If the patient is weak, there may be a spontaneous outbreak of sweating.

3. If the joints do not open with relative ease, the focus should be sought in the corresponding vertical body zone of the head and neck. It may lie in either the jaw, the teeth, or the sinuses, and is either a scar or a chronic infection.

Immediately after concluding the first reflex zone massage of the feet, the *relevant findings* should be noted down, to serve as a reminder for the succeeding treatments. This does not preclude the therapist from adapting to any altered findings she may encounter in the feet during subsequent massages, and by taking into account changes as they occur she will prevent the therapy from becoming a merely routine procedure. Far more important than the static picture given in previously made notes is a *new awareness* of the present state of the patient, which will be reflected on the feet at each visit. New findings should be recorded and added to the basic first history.

Each treatment session is governed by a basic set of rules, but it should gradually be elevated from an exercise of purely technical proficiency to truly creative work.

8.

REACTIONS

At the commencement of therapy, the patient must be fully informed of the meaning and purpose of any reactions which may occur, by means of either a short introductory talk or a suitably prepared pamphlet, such as is used in the training school. If this step is neglected, the patient will misinterpret the reactions and may feel frightened by them.

Any change from the previous state of health, whether pleasant or disturbing, of shorter or longer duration, sharp or stimulating, is an indication of the inner healing capacity of the patient playing its part, and shows that the breaking down and elimination of metabolites and toxins has begun.

Recognition and perception of the differing *forms* and *intensity* of reactions gives those who perform the treatment a worth-while lesson in observation, and shows the need to adapt one's massage to make it more versatile. The therapist must always bear in mind that the sick person is constantly changing — and with him, his disease picture! As practice proceeds the therapist will need to change and modify her therapy and its practical application so that it is always in tune with each new situation. She must be able to alter with the altered needs of each patient. A standard, unchanging performance lacks vitality and becomes stale, and in time ceases to be beneficial.

Note: Chronic illness cannot be *directly* steered towards the healing process. A regenerative detour which is guided by the more or less evident acute phases of such reactions must be sought.

A number of reactions may accompany reflex zone massage, and they are divided into *two main groups:*

(a) *Reactions which occur during reflex zone massage* enable you to observe and assess the immediate tolerance and capacity of the patient, and allow you to graduate *dosage,* intensity and duration of the treatment accordingly. Reactions which can be observed by the therapist include:

1. Changes of expression;

2. Sighing, groaning, whimpering, laughing, etc;

3. Gestures of pain, disquiet or fear.

4. Visible contraction of different muscle groups, which may affect the whole body.

Reaction which may be experienced by the patient include:

1. A spontanous and perhaps profuse outbreak of *sweat* on the palms of the hands. Form this you will know that the patient will respond in a labile and hypersensitive manner to treatment.

2. Alternatively, there may be *enhanced sweating* of the palms, in addition to outbreaks of sweat on particular *areas* or *segments* of the skin (cutaneo-visceral irritability), or over the whole body.

3. A sensation of being *cool* or *chilled*, which begins at the extremities and may penetrate to the central core of the person.

Important: Chilliness is a sign that the capacity of the patient to benefit from treatment has been **exceeded**. Apparently the blood supply to the periphery becomes inadequate — the first indication of shock.

4. Very occasionally the patient experiences an *inner shivering*, which in extreme cases proceeds to *chattering of the teeth*, *tetanus-like spasms* and *circulatory collapse.*

All these types of reaction are indicators of the personal vitality of the patient, and they demand a constant, watchful, vigilant and alert response on the part of the therapist, whose concern must be to avoid reactions which are so strong that they overwhelm the resilience of the patient. This does not mean that should any of the above-mentioned reactions occur, treatment should be interrupted or concluded. They will, however, be factors which influence the intensity and duration of each respective reflex zone massage to the feet. The rule is that you work up to the level of the pain threshold, which varies so widely with each individual. The art of the good therapist lies in finding the right and harmonious balance between his or her strength and dexterity, and the capacity of the patient to benefit from this offering.

If the patient responds to careful and accurately gauged treatment with unexpectedly strong reactions, the following measures will restore and balance the energy of the patient.

First Aid Measures

(i) Remain calm and observant! A therapist who is anxious and tense will aggravate the condition of the patient and transmit her feelings of uncertainty.

(ii) Remember and observe the Arndt-Schultz rule: 'Weak stimuli are beneficial, strong stimuli are detrimental, very strong stimuli are harmful'.

(iii) Taking the heels in the palms of your hands, apply gentle traction to the legs. This will help to regulate the breathing. Ensure that you have a cushion or support under the knees — this will prevent the three dimensional *stretching* from becoming a two dimensional *pulling*.

(iv) Gently stimulate the reflex zone to the solar plexus (which is also the diaphragm) and the heart.

(v) Apply light pressure to (and thereby regulate) the reflex zones of the following endocrine glands: the pituitary gland (which influences the activity of all the other endocrine glands); the parathyroid glands, which share the same reflex zone as the thyroid gland (and regulate the blood calcium levels); the adrenal glands (which govern the secretion of adrenalin).

It is seldom necessary to apply the measures advocated in (v) above, as the patient usually recovers swiftly when breathing and heart rate have returned to normal. Should the patient later feel cool, cold, or start shivering, then passive warming by covering with woollen blankets or hot water bottles is necessary. The calm, warm hands of the therapist are also effective in this warming process when placed against the soles of the feet, or if used to enfold the feet, so that the patient actually feels him or herself to be 'in good hands'.

In such a case, no further treatment is carried out. The patient is left warmly covered, undisturbed, and closely but unobtrusively observed, until there is complete recovery. There is an inner, self-healing capacity present within every single person, which will work to heal the patient in combination with your treatment.

(b) Reactions occuring in the intervals between treatments are an indication of the effects of each reflex zone massage to the feet, specific to each individual patient, and are varied in nature. They generally appear between the second and sixth treatment, and usually last for a few days. There are, of course, patients who will have one or more reactions after the first treatment, and conversely, others who will not experience them until after the eighth or tenth treatment.

As long as treatment of the reflex zone is maintained at the threshold of the proper stimulus, any reactions which occur between treatments should be regarded as desirable and anticipated signs of *healing*. They show the capacity of the body for self-regeneration. This holds true whether they involve temporary *discomfort* or if they are accompanied by *pain*. They reflect an accurate picture of the patient's past and present disease picture.

When extreme reactions to treatment prevail, the patient can be built up by either: very carefully regulating the dosage, intensity and duration of treatment at the next visit, or by omitting the following treatment session. This will give the organism enough time and opportunity for healing regeneration.

The diverse forms which the reactions may take in the intervals between treatments is closely bound to the respective person and the history of his disease. However, apart from this consideration, usually one or more reactions may occur, such as

(i) The patients find themselves deeply *relaxed*. *Sleep* become calmer and deeper. Mental and physical *vitality* improve. Conversely, sleep may become disturbed for a while, and dreams may be more frequent.

(ii) There is a marked increase in the activity of the *skin*, with increased perspiration, which is sometimes malodorous. Occasionally a rash or pustules appear, and very occasionally a boil may erupt. Skin and tissues tonus may improve considerably, so that the whole appearance is of better health and circulation.

(iii) The *kidneys* secrete more urine. The urine may become cloudy, with an unpleasant smell, and if left to stand for some time may develop a heavy sediment.

(iv) *Stools* are increased in bulk, volume and frequency, and also develop an unpleasant smell sometimes. Their mucous content may be increased and they may be unusually discoloured. There is frequently an increase in *flatulence*.

(v) Increase in *secretions* of the mucous membranes of the *nose*, *pharynx* and *bronchi*, which marks a cleansing process. The secretions may vary in colour, odour and consistency.

(vi) *Vaginal discharge* may occur in women, and at times this may be so acid, concentrated and irritating that there is inflammation and pain in the surrounding tissue.

(vii) There may be a brief episode of *fever*. In general, this should be interpreted as a natural mobilization of the defences of the body against disease, and not as a sign of illness.

(viii) *Infected foci in the teeth* may become painful, as may old, poorly healed *scar* tissue, which may also produce an exudate.

(ix) *Previous diseases* which have been suppressed in the past and never truly healed may flare up for a short while. In rare instances a whole range of past illnesses reappear for a short term before complete healing is induced. (Dr H. Reckweg).[9]

(x) *Emotional or psychological unease* may be expressed in a wide range of forms, from weeping to frank discussion of problems.

According to Paracelsus it is Nature or the 'inner doctor' which ordains that the *organs of excretion* are the main vehicle by means of which the body is relieved of stored up toxins and metabolites, some of which may have been present for many years.

It goes without saying that reactions which give rise to the *suspicion of serious illness* must be made known to the doctor.

Responsible therapists know the boundaries and limits of their practice. It is the mark of regard for their profession that, when in doubt, they will seek medical advice once too often rather than too little. In this way, the therapist also becomes more certain of the ranges of her branch of therapy between which she may move, and retains the trust and confidence of her patients.

9.

COMMON CAUSES OF FOOT COMPLAINTS

The following wide range of external and internal causes may give rise to disorders on the feet. Whether or not, and under what circumstances, these lead to abnormality of the underlying reflex zones depends on the *intensity* and *duration* of the stimulus, and upon the *vitality* of the person concerned.

(i) *Overexertion.* (Walking, hiking, strenuous sport carried to extremes.)

(ii) *Fatigue and exhaustion.* (This includes those occupations which necessitate standing all day, expecially on concrete floors, etc.)

(iii) *Immediate injuries.* (Wounds, cuts, perforating or penetrating foreign objects, stings, fractures, sprains.)

(iv) *Inherited dispositions.* (Weakness of the connective tissue; flat, splay feet; T.E. Valgus or T.E. Varus.)

(v) *General circulatory disturbances.* (Varicose veins, varicose ulcers, ulcus cruris, Buerger's disease, intermittent claudication, etc.)

(vi) *Rheumatoid disease,* widespread or localized, which may manifest itself in the feet (e.g. 'arthritic toes').

Even when no direct conclusions may be drawn from the correlation of disturbed reflex zones and deformity on the feet, such deformities always reflect a weakness and impairment which should be noted in your general findings.

10.

SPECIAL OBSERVATIONS TO BE MADE ON THE FEET

The therapist gains an overall impression of the feet in two ways:

(i) *Through palpation* — discussed earlier under 'the grip-sequence'.

(ii) *Through visual observation* and examination. Visual examination is complementary to and enhances the impression gained from physical palpation. No valid, objective conclusions can be drawn with regard to the patient's complaints from visual examination alone.

Note: The beginner must first learn to observe the total surfaces of the feet; she must then have patience, and learn to palpate and observe the smaller surface areas of the feet upon which she is working. It will soon be appreciated that although every foot has the *same* basic anatomical structure, more importantly, each bears entirely *personal and noteworthy characteristics*. For this reason, working with the feet is never boring or monotonous, for the therapist approaches with interest the individual picture of the person engraved on their feet, and perceives the result of her endeavours in the reactions which follow.

Visual Examination
Any departure from the normal in colour, shape, tissue turgor or temperature evident in the appearance of the feet which persists for longer than a few weeks may be the external expression of a disturbed reflex zone. Visual examination includes the following:

(a) The *bony* structure;

(b)   The condition of the *tissues*;

(c)   The condition of the *skin*.

(a) Visual examination of the bony structure of the feet

The importance of the feet as arched structures, bearing the weight of the whole body, is well known and used by many other physical therapy disciplines, including orthopaedic practitioners and chiropractors. They view the foot principally from the perspective of its *dynamic equilibrium*. This approach, although from a different angle, complements and enhances our knowledge when practising reflex zone therapy of the feet.

Thus: changes in the skeletal structure of the feet mean that there is, at the same time, disturbance in the energy distribution within the reflex zones. It follows, therefore, that there is a relationship between any *alteration of the normal alignment of the bony structure* of the feet and a *disorder in corresponding organs* of the body.

Examples:

(i)   A flattened, splayed transverse arch can affect the reflex zone to the shoulder girdle and organs of respiration, and/or the liver gall-bladder on the right foot, the heart on the left.

(ii)   Fallen arches or flat feet can affect the reflex zones to the spinal column.

(iii)   Hallux valgus has its effect upon the reflex zones to the cervical spine and the thyroid gland.

(iv)   Hammer and other deformities of the toes burden all the reflex zones to the head and also the teeth.

(v)   Mycotically infected toenails (onychomycosis) or those which are noticeably different from the normal in shape and texture (wooden nails) indicate that the reflex zones to the head have been in some way affected.

(vi)   Injury or congestion around the inner and outer malleoli and of the heel are united with disorders of the pelvis and hip joints.

(vii) Sunken cuneiform bones imply disease of the intestine.

(b) Visual examination of tissue tonus
The feet show any lymphatic congestion and oedema (pitting oedema) primarily in the region of the ankle, around the malleoli, Achilles tendon, and above the bases of the toe joints on the dorsum of the feet. These are the reflex zones to the pelvis and organs of the upper thorax.
Note: Oedema around the malleoli may in general be attributed to a disorder of the kidneys, heart or circulation. We have also found such patients have considerble congestion in the pelvis, which may be of venous, arterial, lymphatic, nervous system or hormonal origin. There is without doubt an associated disturbance of circulation but this is secondary.
   Diseases of the *heart* and *circulation* are frequently evident to the therapist whilst making a *visual* examination, appearing as tiny pads round the base of the toes on the *left* dorsum.

(c) Visual examination of the skin
The skin of most people's feet is rough and neglected. It is therefore an excellent source of information when visually examined. The type of abnormality or deformity which appears on the feet is not particularly relevant, what is far more important is its *site.*

Example:
A corn at the metatarso-phalangeal joint of the small toe on the left foot reflects some injury to the shoulder. A corn between the right second and third toes bears on the reflex zone to the right eye. Whether a corn, a callous or a mycotic infection (such as athlete's foot) appears over the reflex zone is less important than the visible alteration in the condition of the skin, indicating as it does that the reflex zone to the shoulder or the eye may be affected.
   The skin of the feet is examined for the following *abnormalities:* cracks and crevisses; warts and fissures in the webs between the toes; dull, cold or throbbing skin; athlete's foot; wounds, corns or blisters; heat rash, varicose veins or odour; pigmentation, reddening, desquamation, sweating of the feet, pustules, pimples, vesicles, ulcers; horniness, indentations, puffiness, scars; as well as the shape, colour and texture of each individual toe-nail.
Note: Varicose veins which lie in the vicinity of any of the reflex zones, that is to say on the lower third of the leg between the knee

and ankle joints, should be avoided during reflex zone massage. The same is true for ulcers in this area.

Although a variety of different external factors, (tight shoes, socks, stockings, athlete's foot, fashionably high but unhealthy shoes, footwear made of unsuitable materials, or inadequate personal hygiene) may account for such abnormalities, they are not often the true cause. They frequently encounter a *favourable milieu* for their development because of some inherent *weakness* or predisposition to weakness in the reflex zone over which they appear. In other words there was in these areas an *internal debilitation* present in many cases before the *external disorder* arose.

Example:
Athlete's foot rarely extends over the entire foot, and does not often even affect all the webs between the toes if one has been exposed to infection at a swimming pool or sauna bath. It is typically observed in a specific site, which nearly always coincides with overtaxation of the related organ. Even though the patient does not complain of and may not be aware of dysfunction of an organ or system in his body, this does not mean the absence of disease. He believes, erroneously, that the absence of pain and lack of awareness of the disordered function of his own body is synonymous with health. Athlete's foot is often highly resistant to any form of external treatment, and only heals completely when local external treatment gives rise to a changed and restored internal conditon. Reflex zone massage of the feet is appropriate to bringing about this restoration.
Note: Therapy is not carried out over the areas infected by any fungus. It is directed from healthy tissues towards the diseased parts, but only as far as is hygienically acceptable or tolerable for the patient.

By repeated treatments the circulation to this affected area of skin is improved at the periphery and inwardly. This decreases the perimeter in which the micro-organisms can flourish. A sound and healthy foot would rapidly overcome infection by local application of fungicides or by careful attention to that area. Only when the underlying reflex zone is disordered will such infections thrive.

The *chiropodist*, who must complete an intensive training in some European countries, is for the therapist an invaluable colleague, particularly when he or she has learned and assimilated the principles of reflex zone therapy to the feet.

Whilst the chiropodist may not embark on any therapy, (that is, he may not treat any disease in patients), he will nevertheless treat the feet sensitively, and maintain them in the best possible condition. To this end, corns and callouses are pared away, nails are cut and shaped and ingrowing toenails are prevented.

Because the visual examination is so important, and the source of so much information for the therapist, if is preferable for the patient to visit the chiropodist *after* the first reflex zone massage rather than beforehand.

11.

THE SUBJECTIVE EFFECTS OF REFLEX ZONE THERAPY

The probing hand of the therapist invokes an impulse in the nerve endings of the feet. The result of this in a healthy reflex zone with good circulation is no different from that of a similar tissue displacement in any other healthy part of the body. *It should not be painful.*

When the reflex zone is abnormal, however, the patient reacts to the impulse of pressure, no matter how carefully graduated, simply because it causes pain.

There are distinct grades to the *quality of this pain:*

(i) The most surprising sensation is that of a *sharp, pricking pain,* usually concentrated in an area the size of a pin-head, and often so intensive that the patient wishes to know if it was made by a sharp object or a finger-nail. This pain is usually experienced in the toes and heels.

(ii) The pain which is experienced in the tissues is frequently felt over a *broad area,* and it is not uncommon to hear this pain described as 'pain which is accompanied by a sense of well-being'.

(iii) Exceedingly *sharp* pain is experienced in the webs of the toes or on the lateral aspect of the fifth metatarsal bones, usually in association with the 'milking' or 'wringing' movements used here.

Healthy tissue possesses *good tonus.* Painful responses to treatment should be regarded as a warning signal. According to Dr R. Voll, pain is 'the crying out of the tissues for a free flow of energy'.[10]

Do not confuse the *subjective* accounts of ailments by the

patient with your own *objective* findings resulting from *visual* and *physical examination*, for the following reasons:

(a)   The patient is describing a solitary symptom;

(b)   He sometimes forgets the essentials and emphasizes the less essential;

(c)   He mentions none of his latent problems, since he is as yet unaware of them;

(d)   Because of severe afflictions in a particular organ or system, pain which is less acute or troublesome in other places or symptoms which are less troublesome are often glossed over. These first come to light when the initial strong pain has diminished in quality. So patients believe over and over again that the therapy 'makes them sicker than they were before', when in the treatment sequence they become aware of pain which had previously been overborne because it had not impinged so strongly.

Most patients believe that their illness commenced with the first appearance of the first symptoms. 'Yesterday evening I caught a cold'; 'On Sunday the rheumatism in my shoulder started playing up'; 'Since I developed the colic I've had gall-bladder problems'. This is not the truth of the matter. Every illness is preceded by a *prodromal* or *incubation* period, which may last for days, weeks, months or years. Only when the patient cannot successfully maintain homeostasis from within does the acute and then later the chronic phase of the illness become apparent. It is only in *accidents* that injury and signs and symptoms occur simultaneously.

The beginner will find it difficult at times not to attach more importance to what the patient says than to what she has discovered as a result of her own examination. From the very first reflex zone massage to the feet she must practise *self-reliance*, and will in due course become independent of the subjective statements made by her patients.

Example:
The patient complains of some stomach disorder, and believes that he is otherwise 'quite healthy'. Objective palpation of the feet, however, reveals that as well as the stomach, the small

intestine, the liver, the cervical spine, the solar plexus and the right knee respond abnormally in their reflex zones. If the therapist is uncertain of her ground, she will not know which finding is correct. In every case, *visual* and *palpable observations* arising from your examination are more valid than any mention of *symptoms*, and the treatment will then not be directed toward an isolated illness, but to the *sick person in his entirety, in all his aspects*.

12.
INTERPRETATION OF ABNORMAL REFLEX ZONES

When visual and palpable examination of the feet confirm that an abnormal reflex zone is present, then a corresponding disorder may be discovered in the related organ or system *at the moment of treatment*.

This finding is insufficient to determine the *cause*, the *type* or the *duration* of this disorder. A diversity of influences may lie in the background, of which the following are but examples:

(i) *Overtiredness* such as pain at the base of the spine after a long car journey.

(ii) *Over-exertion* — e.g. strain on the heart after strenuous sport, or a brain which is overtaxed after long hours of study.

(iii) *Latent disease,* whose symptoms have not yet become apparent. The disturbed reflex zone may warn of such disease, and react abnormally in patients who are not as yet aware of illness. In this case reflex zones are are found to be painful some days before an infection of the throat, and weeks before painful limitation of the shoulder joint makes itself felt.

(iv) *Acute disease processes* — such as acute otitis media, acute gastritis and acute nephritis.

(v) *Chronic disease processes* — such as chronic bronchitis, emphysema, tumours and myocardial infirmity.

(vi) *Hyperactivity* of an organ — for example hyperthyroidism.

(vii) *Hypoactivity* of an organ — hypo and achlorhydria of the stomach, hormonal deficiences.

(viii) *Palsy*, atrophy, atony, degeneration — as in prolapsed uterus or rectum, floating kidneys, arthroses.

(ix)   *Inherited predisposition* to disease — which may include genetic tendencies to skeletal or connective tissue weaknesses, allergies, inherited disorders.

(x)   *Accidents* — fractures, sprains, bruises, injuries.

It will be seen from the above list that the cause of an abnormal reflex zone is not always a 'crystalline deposit'. (E. Ingham).[4,5]

There is as yet no scientific explanation which has been substantiated for the manifestation of painful reflex zones, no matter whether they appear within less than a second (as in the case of accidents), or are built up over many months (as in chronic illness). We have, until now, considered it from the angle of a functional Energy failing, and recognize hyper, hypo or atonus in the tissues of the feet, and are speaking in this context of an energy stream which is not physiological, but is perceptible in the tissues as an energy fullness, an energy deficiency or an energy absence.

In the framework of these disorders there may frequently occur a secondary deposition which may take many forms, as for example uric acid crystals, as was decribed many times by E. Ingham in her writings. For the reason described above, the therapist will refrain from rash 'diagnosis' which may need subsequent revision.

It must further be mentioned that in patients who are gravely ill, disturbed psychologically, and in many who are terminally ill with cancer (particularly when they are having cobalt treatment), that reflex zone massage of the feet does not always give an exact picture of the physical condition of the patient at that time. It may also be quite possible that infirmity of an organ is not only to be perceived in a reflex zone, but may even prefer to leave another 'signature', in for example the connective tissue or the meridians of acupuncture.

Nevertheless, the information which an abnormal reflex zone affords is very useful in the *differential diagnosis* of numerous illnesses which have not been clarified in other medical systems.

Example:
In acute abdominal illness the reflex zones to the kidneys, gall-bladder, appendix, stomach and ovaries are easier to distinguish

on the feet than the organs in the abdomen, and they usually react sensitively to pressure.

13.

COURSE OF TREATMENT WITH REFLEX ZONE THERAPY

The number of reflex zone massages to the feet which will be necessary for each individual patient cannot be determined or stated with exactitude at the commencement of treatment. The patient's background and the immediate general condition of the whole organism is too complex to allow this.

Any of the following factors may influence the condition:

(i)   Climatic stimuli, (gale force winds or the commencement of cold or wet weather).

(ii)   Changes of diet, (whether while travelling, or at official dinners, or highly spiced and seasoned foods tried experimentally or occasionally).

(iii)   Alterations in the waking-sleeping rhythm (night duty, shift work, anxiety and over-excitement).

(iv)   The continual changes in the personal biorhythms from the active to the passive phase and vice versa.

(v)   Latent illness, a quiescent phase or the incubation period of an infectious disease.

(vi)   Psychic or emotional trauma in the family or at work.

(vii)   Geographical areas where geopathic stimuli exert a strong influence, or from the mechanization of the environment, either in one's place of work or the home. Consider the prevalence of radios, digital alarm clocks and watches, television, too many mirrors and plastic or synthetic fabrics.

(viii) Poisons in the air, water, polishing and washing up liquids and sprays, in food, in synthetic fabrics or impregnated in dusters and cleaning and polishing cloths, (even in catgut sutures).

Rules for Treatment

As long as positive reactions result from your treatment, there is value in continuing that treatment. This hold true even when an average of *10 - 12 treatments*, at best given two or three times a week, has been completed.

The number of treatments needed depends in the first instance on the *nature of illness,* the *competent ability of the body* to react to treatment, on the *vitality* and *inner adjustment* of the patient, the *biological age* and the manner in which the patient conducts his or her life.

Not infrequently a single reflex zone massage to the feet restores to essential order dysfunction of some years standing. When this happens it does not mean that the treatment should be discontinued, as a short series of foot treatments will have the effect of stabilizing and consolidating that person's conditon.

When no particular disorder is apparent, a short course of treatment can be repeated after an interval of a year or so, or whenever the patient feels it to be necessary.

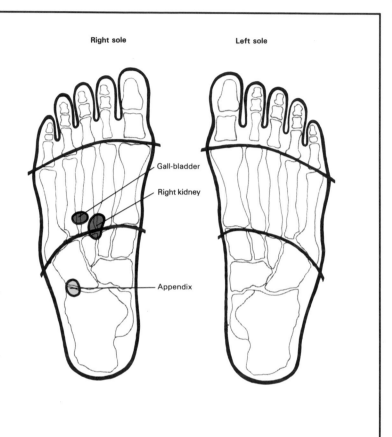

Right sole   Left sole

Gall-bladder

Right kidney

Appendix

Diagram 12:   Differential Diagnosis in Abdominal Disease

Left dorsum   Right dorsum

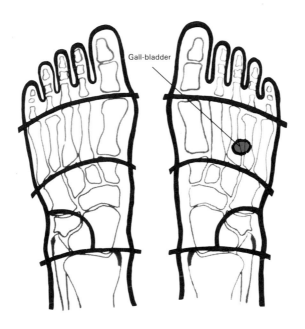

Gall-bladder

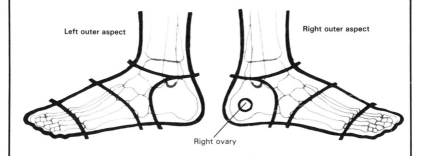

Left outer aspect   Right outer aspect

Right ovary

14.

TREATMENT COMBINATIONS

When reflex zone therapy to the feet does not fully produce the desired improvement in the patient's condition it may be necessary to use another form of treatment as well. Reflex zone massage to the feet is a natural therapy. It may therefore be allied to other similar natural healing disciplines for enhancement.

Combinations which may *increase* the curative effect are:

1. All *naturopathic* health rules, which encourage detoxification of the body fluids, especially the blood and lymphatic fluid. These include the regime of fasting for health and in order to improve intestinal function, as advocated by Dr F.X. Mayr[11]; mild abstinence[12] and fasting according to the rules laid sown by Schroth and Felke and by Buchinger.

2. *Hydrotherapy* — as advocated by Kneipp[6], Kuhne[13], Priessnitz and Schlenz.

3. Similar proven *manual therapies* — acumassage, connective tissue massage[1,2], chiropractic and chirogymnastics, classical massage, manual lymph drainage and shiatsu.[24]

4. *Herbal* and *homoeopathic* remedies, *acupuncture*.

5. *Dietetic* measures such as those advocated by Bircher-Benner, Bruker, Cousa, Evers, Hay[15], F.X. Mayr, Waerland.

6. Deep *breathing* exercises, *gymnastics*, *postural correction* according to Alexander[21, 22], Middendorf, Schaarschuch[16], Schlaffhorst-Andersen and Schroth (for treatment of scoliosis).

7.   Treatment of a *disordered energy field*.
(a) Treatment of *scars* through *neural therapy*.
(b) Treatment of infective foci in *teeth* and *sinuses* without recourse to chemical treatments using proven biochemical methods.
(c) Eliminating *'geopathic'* irritations and stimuli from the places where one works and lives. An excess of cement, steel, glass and artificial fibres[27] creates an atmosphere which is antipathetic to healthy living.

Note: Reflex zone massage to the feet may also act beneficially on a 'disturbed field' which lies outside the feet, such as

(a) *Scars.* Patients often mention that during or after a reflex zone massage they feel a prickling, pulling or light stabbing sensation in a scar. It is a fairly common occurrence that reflex zone massage to an area of the feet which corresponds to a part of the body which bears a scar, brings about a spontaneous haematoma over or around such scar tissue. As the haematoma reabsorbs, any pain and contraction of the scar which was felt prior to treatment is diminished.

(b) *Teeth.* Granulomas, abscesses, osteitis (bone infection) and parotitis can be effectively treated when the tooth itself is still vital (that is if there has been no root treatment). Nevertheless, in such cases it is essential to co-operate with a qualified dentist.
Special *care* is needed when treating people with *old injuries* sustained during the war! Grenade and shell splinters which have become encapsulated in any organ or tissue may, as a result of reflex zone massage to the feet move from their previous fixed position.
When a combination of treatments is being carried out, they must be co-ordinated with one another. It is dangerous for therapeutic stimuli to follow one another too quickly, and the effect of one may cancel out the effect of another.
If a warm footbath has been taken immediately *before* reflex zone massage, the observations which you make visually and as a result of palpation will be distorted due to recent thorough warming, particularly if chemical bath salts have been added to the water. If passive warming of the feet is necessary, it is best done at the end of treatment.
Less effective, even harmful, is the *indiscriminate use* of the

different *grips* to unselected areas of the feet. Use firm discipline in confining, restricting and limiting yourself to only that which is effective. Anyone wishing to employ more than one manual therapy discipline in a single treatment must indeed know what he is doing!

15.
EMOLLIENTS AND 'FOOT AIDS'

No emollient should be used when practising reflex zone massage to the feet. The therapist may apply a herbal ointment, oil, or an aetheric oil with healing properties in order to stimulate the circulation at the *end* of treatment.

Beware of chemical footsprays! They clog the pores and prevent the feet from being able to rid themselves and the body of excretions from the sweat glands. Suppressing the ability of the body to sweat through the feet is unwise. Excessive sweating, particularly if malodorous, is an indication of imbalance which should be heeded.

Note: The therapist may gather much valuable information from patients who present with different, strange odours given off by the feet. If they are markedly offensive during treatment a pure cologne water may be applied. The patient should be informed that shoes, socks and stockings of synthetic materials increase the likelihood of sweating, and because there is no local ventilation, it may become offensive. Daily changes of socks and stockings and daily footbaths (to which sea salt or cider vinegar may be added) are worth-while measures for these patients to take.

'Mechanical Aids' for the Feet

With the proliferation of so-called 'foot aids' such as rollers, mats, spheres, platters made of wood, clay, plastic, metal, rubber and brushes, and partially or wholly electrically operated gadgets, a new type of useless toy has come into being. These articles are used in ignorance of a coherent approach to treating specific disorders.

The use of such implements is not directly harmful, nor is it unprofitable. The propaganda which has been invented to promote their sale has invested them with a great deal of potential which they do not have. Often it is like comparing the inadvertent prick of a finger with a sewing needle with the practice of acupuncture, or wetting of the feet with hydrotherapy, so faintly do such implements invoke a *specific* action. At best they tap the symptoms of the patient.

The use of such aids is therefore only meaningful when they are recognized for what they are. They can promote the circulation and the lymphatic drainage of the feet. They may warm you up, and they may strengthen and relax weakened or taut musculature of the feet and make them more elastic, but only when they are rightly employed, and not when their use is exaggerated.

These implements are nevertheless *no instruments of reflex zone therapy*. This is the realm of the responsible therapist who knows why, where, when, how strongly and for how long to work on the feet.

Example:

Imagine a person with a heart or kidney disorder, in whom disease of these organs has resulted in the corresponding reflex zones of the feet being sensitive. By using one of the above-mentioned implements he could do himself more harm than good. He may not be aware of the first principle of this work — sedate hyperactivity and stimulate flaccidity. In addition to this, moreover, he inevitably finds himself concerned solely with the symptoms rather than broadening his horizon to consider the causes.

16.
CONTRA-INDICATIONS

As with all therapies, reflex zone therapy of the feet has its limits, beyond which its practice is ineffective. Contra-indications to therapy are:

(i)   Acute infectious fevers and diseases.

(ii) Acute inflammations of the venous and lymphatic systems. Deep vein thrombosis.

(iii) Conditions where surgery is indicated.

(iv) Sudeck's atrophy of the feet, gangrene, and extensive mycotic infections of the feet.

(v)   Pregnancies which are unstable or at risk.

(vi) Osteoporosis and decalcification resulting from accidents leading to consequent poor healing or malunion of bone. Possible decalcification resulting from tumours.

Experience has shown that, apart from these, chronic and progressive or terminal illnesses (such as ankylosing spondylitis, multiple sclerosis, Parkinson's disease, cancer and paralysis) will often show a response to treatment of the reflex zones of the feet. The disease may not be amenable to cure, but the patient may often be made more comfortable. The following *improvements* may accompany treatment:

(a) Functional improvement of the organs of *excretion* — the kidneys, intestines, skin and lungs.

(b) Alleviation of *pain*, even in the terminal stages of cancer and during renal dialysis.

(c) Increase in *control* of the sphincter muscles of the bladder and bowels.

Note; Patients in whom recent surgery has resulted in retention of urine may frequently be spared catheterization if the reflex zones to the bladder and solar plexus are treated. This is already being successfully carried out in some hospitals in Europe.

17.
TREATING ONESELF

Anyone who is mobile, whose joints are flexible, and who can easily raise their legs to the level of the trunk can endeavour to treat the reflex zones of their own feet. When this is done, however, there are certain points to remember, particularly when the attempt is made by people who have not been trained in this discipline.

(i) Self treatment is not more than general health care, or a form of first aid, in the same way as one might use Kneipp hydrotherapy at home.

(ii) The influence exerted by the personality of the therapist is absent, as with self treatment one is both patient and therapist at the same time.

(iii) Since, of necessity, one must raise one's feet, relaxation is difficult to achieve.

(iv) The characteristic features indicating that adequate treatment has been given (sweating, coolness, inner warmth) cannot be assessed objectively. Sweating may be the result of the exertion of self treatment rather than from having correctly measured the dosage required. It is also difficult to observe cooling of one's own extremities.

(v) Hands which are unpractised soon tire. Implements such as wooden pestles, rubber mats or vibrators give no clue to the differing state of tissue tonus in the feet.

(vi) Anyone who is inexperienced or inexpert in observing the progress of disease is unable to assess the reaction phase correctly. They are inclined to lay undue emphasis on looked for reactions, and to minimize (through ignorance) the actual state of the disease, which is truly the province of the doctor. They are usually swayed by the obvious symptoms because they do not understand the interaction of all systems.

(vii) The initial enthusiasm of people when first coming into contact with this interesting method often falls into one of two extremes:
(a) resignation and outright condemnation when it does not always and immediately offer relief; or
(b) fanaticism, which breeds the little 'wonder doctor', who instantly markets a diagnosis and gives advice which is presented as a total and instant cure.

Notwithstanding the above, good self treatment is preferable to bad treatment from a therapist.
The ideal working team would consist of:

- A well informed and interested doctor, who not only assigns patients to you but will oversee their treatment as well.

- A responsible therapist, who has been well schooled in practice and theory, and has insight into the constantly changing circumstances of the patient's life.

- A competent, conscientious chiropodist.

- A patient who is open-minded and willing to give the benefit of the doubt to a treatment of which he knows nothing, and prepared to co-operate.

18.
THE 'RIGHT AGE' FOR REFLEX ZONE MASSAGE

Over and over again one hears that those over the age of seventy and children under the age of three or four years are advised against having this treatment. The argument which is advanced is that they will not easily be able to bear the pain of reflex zone therapy. What is overlooked is that it is not the treatment which 'gives' them pain. Pain is not an abstract quality. It has already assumed a personal quality by being present in a sick person. As far as the therapy is concerned, the individual pain threshold is readily discerned through the reactions which manifest during treatment. Every sick person, regardless of age, suffers from that pain which directly relates to his illness and must be physically and emotionally endured. A responsible therapist will not overreach the tolerance of the patient's pain threshold, and will work within these highly personal limits.

Years of practical experience have shown that *elderly people* who are responsive to this form of therapy will respond amazingly quickly and positively to natural healing stimuli. Often their regenerative ability is as good as if not better than that of younger people, who have had greater exposure to environmental and nutritional pollution. As most people in the West enjoy a materially higher standard of living today than in previous decades, it is even more imperative that they should be well cared for in their old age, so that they may pass the remainder of their lifespan relatively free of affliction, and that they can depend on their own strength. Even when no acute infirmity lies ahead of them one or two courses of reflex zone massage each year is an appropriate prophylactic measure for both the young and the elderly.

As far as the treatment of *children* is concerned, they cannot accurately describe experience. They must, from birth, learn to cope with and bear disagreeable stimuli from their surroundings. Thus, a reflex zone massage to the feet may be given in the first few days of life. Sucklings and children are grateful patients. Most of them have a more uncomplicated understanding of healing pain than adults, and are far less demanding than their over-indulged elders realize.

Over the years, many interesting observations have been made regarding children. Even those who are relatively healthy and free of ailments often manifest abnormal zones on their feet where one least expects to find them. The explanation is only found when visual and palpable examination of the parents feet is made. Painful reflex zones of the feet of parents and their offspring display an amazing '*inherited disposition*' to an illness. The inference is that such inherited predispositions are already evident in childhood, and may be amenable to treatment by massage of the reflex zones of the feet at that time.

A prominent finding is increased sensitivity in the lymphatic reflex zones of the feet. This is presumably in part due to faulty diet. Mother finds it troublesome to breastfeed her infant, and in many cases dismisses it as being old-fashioned. Later on, products made up of white refined flour and sugar form too great a proportion of the child's daily nutrition. In addition, the repeated administration of proprietary medicines instead of healing remedies and too many immunizations also play their part. It is in precisely such children with weakened resistance that reflex zone massage is effective in stimulating and building them up.

19.
FEET AND HANDS

A legitimate question is frequently asked: Why do most therapists (including Dr Fitzgerald and Eunice Ingham) concern themselves more with the feet than the hands? According to the ten zone division of the body it should in theory be possible to perform the same therapy on the hands. Besides which, the hands are better cared for than the feet, they are more accessible for treatment, and, as can be seen from their anatomical structure, they are softer and more flexible.

Despite these apparent advantages, practice in fact dictates unequivocally that treatment is more effective on the feet. Treatment of the feet gives far better therapeutic results than does that of the hands.

Perhaps it is because the total body weight passes through the feet, and they are weighed down by gravity. Thus the feet have a reciprocal connexion with the earth, and they may be imagined as two poles, responsible for the equalization of Man's electromagnetic field. The feet have often been likened to the roots of a plant, which we know have a great capacity for regeneration.

Not without reason did Sebastian Kneipp stress the value of treatment of the feet. Walking on dewy grass, treading in water, vinegar soaked stockings were amongst the treatments he advocated. It is unfortunate that these valuable treatment measures have been neglected.

Also, the effective treatment which has resulted in our experience from the use of the Schiele apparatus (a temperature raising footbath) the Schluter footbaths and, more recently, the remarkably curative results achieved by the French herbalist Maurice Mességué[20] all point in the same direction.

Cold feet have long been incriminated as a predisposing factor in illnesses such as tonsillitis, laryngitis, bronchitis, cystitis, pyelitis and otitis in susceptible people, as well as other acute and chronic ailments.

The healthy stimulus of walking barefooted on the beach or on grass is generally held to be strengthening and beneficial to the circulation of the feet. There is also a growing interest in shoes which do not cramp and confine the feet, such as Kneipp, Berkeman and Birkenstock sandals in Europe, and Nature shoes in England.

When comparing the hands with the feet, we assign to the hands greater importance in relation to the thinking and feeling areas of life. Hands make music, write, caress, pray, model and gesticulate: so that even at the physical level they fulfil a different function to the feet. The feet on the other hand give us the feeling of being 'grounded', and from the substantial base of the surface of the earth we learn to raise ourselves and walk erectly.

Because they are generally so neglected and ill cared for, the feet respond gratefully to care and treatment, although they are still the orphans of health care. Hands are freer in their movement, which is usually in the element of air, and are usually solicitously cared for and adorned.

Practice has proven that whilst treatment of the reflex zones of the hands is complementary to treatment of the reflex zones of the feet, emphasis should remain on treatment of the reflex zones of the feet. These neglected surfaces may reveal surprising insights into the open secret of the enduring laws of nature and biological renewal.

20.
REFLEX ZONES OF
THE NERVOUS SYSTEM

As a result of continuing studies and a series of trials which we have carried out, we have learned that stimulus can be given not only to organs, bones and muscles, but also to the *nervous system*, whose reflex zones and points are also displayed on the feet.

We started with the discovery and development of a network of reflex zones to the motor nervous system. Today, however, thanks to the personal skill of Walter Froneberg and his dedication to this study, we are also able to identify the reflex zones to the *autonomic nervous system*. This expansion of our fundamental knowledge allows us to use this therapy very specifically in the fields of orthopaedics and neurology. On the one hand we can stimulate the reflex zones of the central nervous system by working on the reflex zones of muscles and joints thus innervated, and on the other hand we can treat malfunction in the autonomic nervous system. As the cause of malfunction of an organ is frequently found in the autonomic nervous system, the discovery of these new reflex zones should prove their worth in helping many conditions, the treatment of which was hitherto uncertain.

The grip-sequence, which has been described earlier, and which is the foundation stone of this work, is not employed when treating the reflex zones of the nervous system. In these cases the disease picture is frequently complicated by infection and stress.

As the treatment of these reflex zones cannot be learnt theoretically, the expanded diagrams showing the reflex zones to the nervous system have not been included in this book. Their description is purposely omitted, and the general information given in the earlier charts (see diagram of the 1976 publication, below) is adequate for any one starting to learn reflex zone massage of the feet.

Because we are responsible both for the method and to our patients, this specialization (which is not entirely without risk in irresponsible hands) is only given in later practical courses of instruction, when therapists have proved their skill in the practice of reflex zone massage to the feet, and have shown thereby that they can benefit responsibly from this advanced stage of practice.

21.
CAUSAL REFLEX ZONES

The concept of Causal Reflex Zones (CRZ) derives from the relationship of each disturbed reflex zone on the feet to the underlying cause (or origin) of the complaint.

There is a distinction drawn between symptomatic and causal treatment. When a *symptomatic* approach is adopted, a patient complaining of pain in the stomach is treated only in the reflex zones to the stomach; one with an aching shoulder is treated only in the shoulder reflex zones, and one with sciatica has treatment confined to the reflex zone at the base of the spine.

When the approach is that of seeking the *cause* of the condition, one is concerned not only with the symptoms, but also with whatever may be the *underlying cause*. In other words, the background is also fully examined. Thus, one may find that in the patient who complains of pain in the stomach the reflex zone to the solar plexus requires treatment as well as that of the stomach; the patient who has limitation of shoulder movement may also have a disorder of the liver or postural changes in the spinal column; and the patient suffering from sciatica should perhaps be attending a urologist or the dentist, because there is a focus of infection there.

It is not necessary to treat all theoretically possible CRZ for every disease picture. Selection depends on the *visual* and *palpable observations* made on the feet of the *individual* patient. When one sees that a reflex zone is abnormal it is treated, otherwise not.

From this follows the fundamental principle that every patient should have *all* the reflex zones tested for their sensitivity, and both visual and palpable examination made at the first reflex zone massage of the feet. Only in this way is the therapist able to build up an objective picture of the initial presenting condition of the patient. This then serves as a guideline for the whole of the

Supplementary Table: Reflex Zones of the Nervous System

Walter Froneberg D-5144 Wegberg-Dalheim

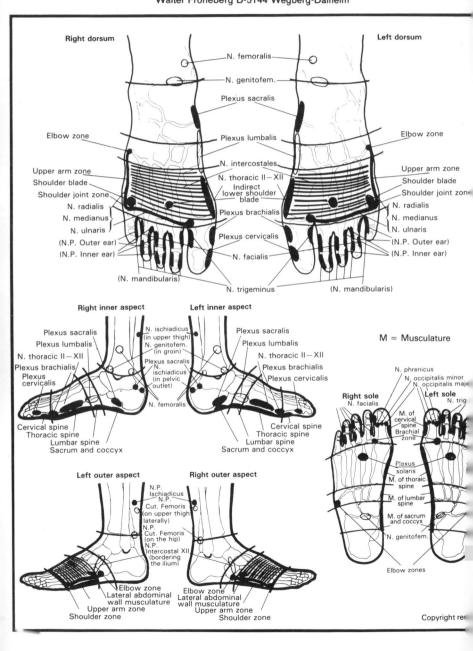

Right dorsum   **Left dorsum**

N. femoralis
N. genitofem.
Plexus sacralis

Elbow zone   Plexus lumbalis   Elbow zone

N. intercostales

Upper arm zone   N. thoracic II—XII   Upper arm zone
Shoulder blade   Indirect   Shoulder blade
Shoulder joint zone   lower shoulder blade   Shoulder joint zone
N. radialis   Plexus brachialis   N. radialis
N. medianus   N. medianus
N. ulnaris   Plexus cervicalis   N. ulnaris
(N.P. Outer ear)   (N.P. Outer ear)
(N.P. Inner ear)   N. facialis   (N.P. Inner ear)

(N. mandibularis)   (N. mandibularis)
N. trigeminus

Right inner aspect   **Left inner aspect**

Plexus sacralis   N. ischiadicus (in upper thigh)   Plexus sacralis
Plexus lumbalis   N. genitofem. (in groin)   Plexus lumbalis
N. thoracic II—XII   Plexus sacralis   N. thoracic II—XII
Plexus brachialis   N. ischiadicus (in pelvic outlet)   Plexus brachialis
Plexus cervicalis   Plexus cervicalis

N. femoralis

Cervical spine   Cervical spine
Thoracic spine   Thoracic spine
Lumbar spine   Lumbar spine
Sacrum and coccyx   Sacrum and coccyx

M = Musculature

N. phrenicus
N. occipitalis minor
N. occipitalis maj[e]

Right sole   **Left sole**
N. facialis   N. trig[

M. of cervical spine
Brachial zone

Plexus solaris
M. of thoracic spine

M. of lumbar spine

M. of sacrum and coccyx

N. genitofem.

Elbow zones

Left outer aspect   **Right outer aspect**

N.P. Ischiadicus
N.P. Cut. Femoris (on upper thigh laterally)
N.P. Cut. Femoris (on the hip)
N.P. Intercostal XII (bordering the ilium)

Elbow zone   Elbow zone
Lateral abdominal wall musculature   Lateral abdominal wall musculature
Upper arm zone   Upper arm zone
Shoulder zone   Shoulder zone

subsequent series of treatments.

Therapy is varied in each successive treatment according to the patient's account of the *nature, duration* and *severity* of reactions which have taken place in the intervals between treatment, but the painful reflex zones take priority in the pattern of treatment which is worked out.

Possible Courses Which Treatment May Take:
A patient presenting with *headache* can be used to illustrate the *variety* of possible causal relationships. For example, seven patients come for therapy complaining of the same symptom, namely headache.

Basic treatment always takes place to the reflex zones of the head, which are the *symptom zones*. The following *causal reflex zones* must be considered:

(i)   The alimentary tract.

(ii) Altered dynamics of the spinal column, particularly in the cervical vertebrae.

(iii) Teeth and sinuses.

(iv) The genito-urinary tract.

(v)   The solar plexus and diaphragm, whose reflex zones may be a factor in conditions of stress and psychic disturbance.

(vi) The organs of respiration.

(vii) A combination of any of the above-mentioned organ reflex zones.

7th Patient with Headache

Basic treatment:	*Causal relationships:*
Reflex zones of the head.	Interconnected systemic disorder:
CRZ:	Alimentary *and* respiratory tracts;
All reflex zones referred to in patients (i) – (vi)	Spiral column *as well as* the teeth and sinuses; Urogenital tract *as well as* autonomic nervous system.

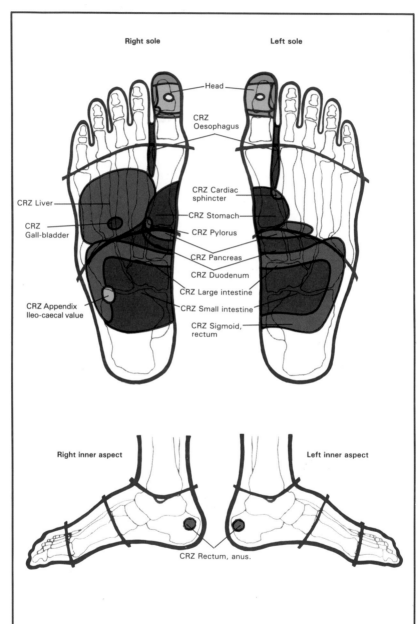

Right sole   Left sole

Head

CRZ Oesophagus

CRZ Cardiac sphincter

CRZ Liver

CRZ Stomach

CRZ Gall-bladder

CRZ Pylorus

CRZ Pancreas

CRZ Duodenum

CRZ Large intestine

CRZ Appendix Ileo-caecal value

CRZ Small intestine

CRZ Sigmoid, rectum

Right inner aspect   Left inner aspect

CRZ Rectum, anus.

Diagram 13: Headache — Synopsis of Related Causes:
Digestive Tract

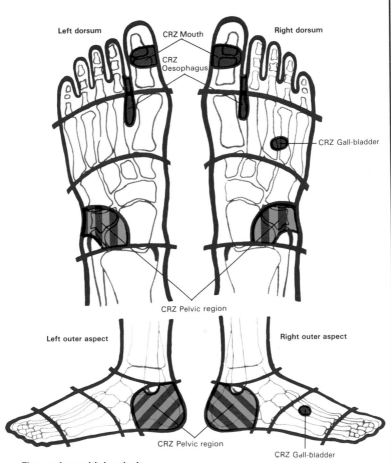

Left dorsum — CRZ Mouth — Right dorsum
CRZ Oesophagus
CRZ Gall-bladder
CRZ Pelvic region

Left outer aspect — Right outer aspect
CRZ Pelvic region
CRZ Gall-bladder

First patient with headache
Related cause:
Digestive tract disorder
Symptoms occur in:
Zones of the head
Causal Reflex Zones (CRZ):
Stomach, cardiac sphincter and pyloric sphincter;
the three segments of the small intestine;
large intestine, particularly the ileo-caecal valve;
(transition from small to large intestine), sigmoid, rectal and anal
areas;
Pancreas; liver and gall-bladder;
Pelvic regions (which share a reflex relationship with organs in the
lower abdomen).

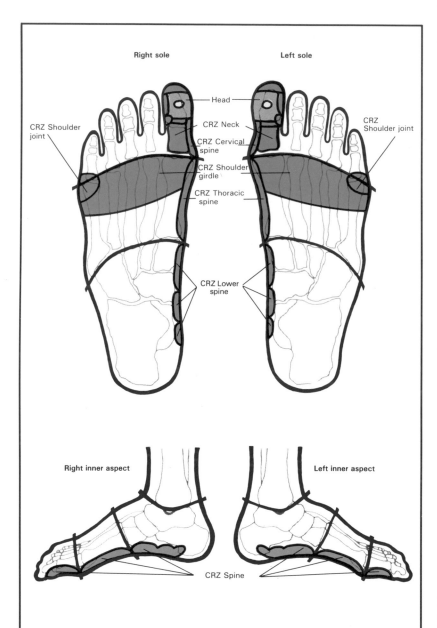

Right sole

Left sole

Head

CRZ Neck

CRZ Cervical spine

CRZ Shoulder girdle

CRZ Thoracic spine

CRZ Shoulder joint

CRZ Shoulder joint

CRZ Lower spine

Right inner aspect

Left inner aspect

CRZ Spine

Diagram 14: Headache — Synopsis of Related Causes: Dynamics of the Vertebral Column and Joints

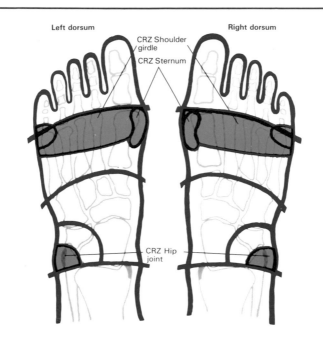

Left dorsum   Right dorsum

CRZ Shoulder girdle

CRZ Sternum

CRZ Hip joint

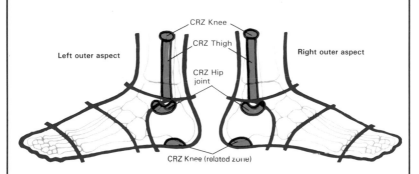

CRZ Knee

CRZ Thigh

Left outer aspect   Right outer aspect

CRZ Hip joint

CRZ Knee (related zone)

Second patient with headache

Related cause:

Disturbed dynamic equilibrium of the vertebral column

Symptoms occur in:

Zones of the head

CRZ: Neck; entire vertebral column, particularly that area where the disorder is most pronounced (usually cervical vertebrae); shoulder gir-dle and shoulder joints; hip joints and knee joints.

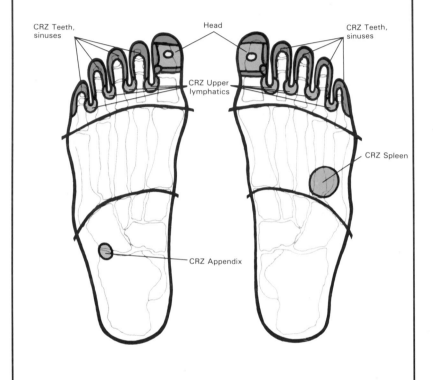

Right sole

Left sole

CRZ Teeth, sinuses

Head

CRZ Teeth, sinuses

CRZ Upper lymphatics

CRZ Spleen

CRZ Appendix

Diagram 15: Headache — Synopsis of Related Causes: Infective Focus in Teeth, Sinuses

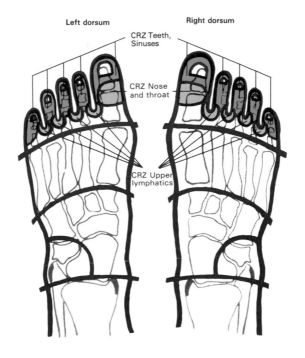

Left dorsum   Right dorsum

CRZ Teeth,
Sinuses

CRZ Nose
and throat

CRZ Upper
lymphatics

Third Patient with Headache:
Causal Relationships:
Area of jaw and teeth
Symptoms occur in:
Zones of the Head
CRZ: Sinuses, teeth;
Nose and throat;
Lymphatic channels of the head and neck;
Spleen (as in all infections),
Appendix

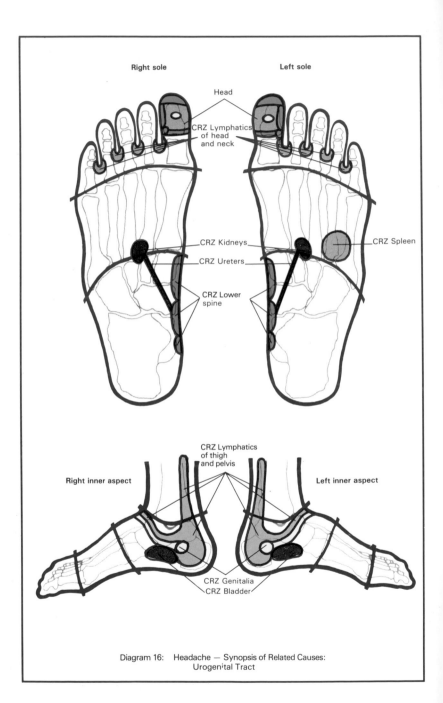

Right sole

Left sole

Head

CRZ Lymphatics of head and neck

CRZ Kidneys

CRZ Spleen

CRZ Ureters

CRZ Lower spine

CRZ Lymphatics of thigh and pelvis

Right inner aspect

Left inner aspect

CRZ Genitalia

CRZ Bladder

Diagram 16:   Headache — Synopsis of Related Causes:
Urogenital Tract

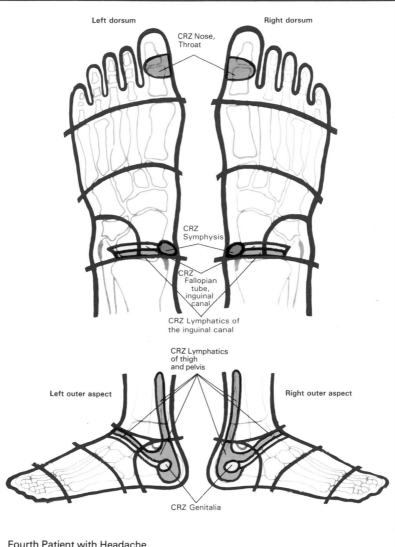

Left dorsum

Right dorsum

CRZ Nose,
Throat

CRZ
Symphysis

CRZ
Fallopian
tube,
inguinal
canal

CRZ Lymphatics of
the inguinal canal

CRZ Lymphatics
of thigh
and pelvis

Left outer aspect

Right outer aspect

CRZ Genitalia

Fourth Patient with Headache
Causal Relationships:
Disease of urogenital tract
Symptoms occur in:
Zones of the head
CRZ: Kidneys, Ureters and bladder; Genitalia; Lymphatic pathways in the
groin and in the head and neck; lower spine; Pelvis and symphysis, spleen

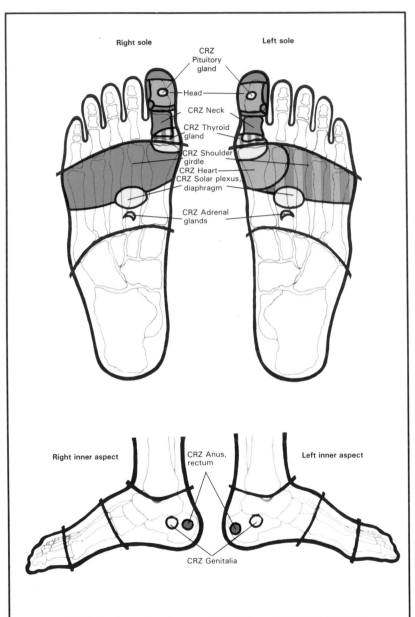

Right sole

Left sole

CRZ Pituitary gland

Head

CRZ Neck

CRZ Thyroid gland

CRZ Shoulder girdle

CRZ Heart

CRZ Solar plexus, diaphragm

CRZ Adrenal glands

Right inner aspect

CRZ Anus, rectum

Left inner aspect

CRZ Genitalia

DIAGRAM 17:   Headache — Synopsis of Related Causes: imbalance in Autonomic
Nervous System, Stress

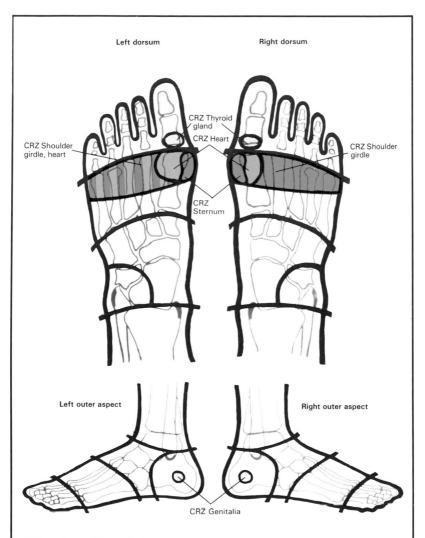

Left dorsum   Right dorsum

CRZ Thyroid gland
CRZ Heart
CRZ Shoulder girdle, heart
CRZ Shoulder girdle
CRZ Sternum

Left outer aspect   Right outer aspect

CRZ Genitalia

Fifth patient with Headache
Causal Relationships:
Disorder of autonomic nervous system, possibly of the psyche; stress.
Symptoms occur in:
Zones of the head.
CRZ: Solar plexus (the same zone as the diaphragm); all endocrine glands:
Pituitary, Thyroid, Adrenal glands, Genitalia; Shoulder girdle, Neck (because
of the "Burden the sick person has to carry on their shoulders"); Heart,
sternum, Spleen.

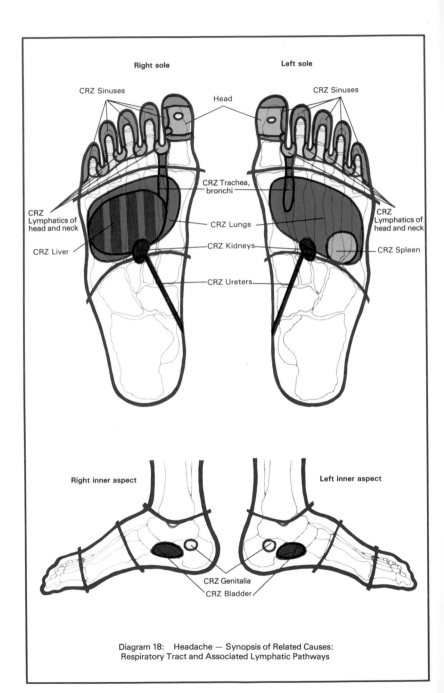

Diagram 18: Headache — Synopsis of Related Causes:
Respiratory Tract and Associated Lymphatic Pathways

Left sole   Right sole

CRZ Sinuses

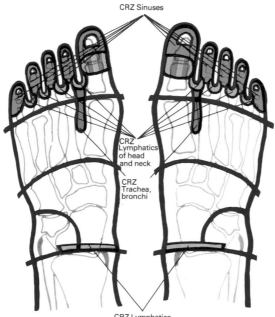

CRZ Lymphatics of head and neck

CRZ Trachea, bronchi

CRZ Lymphatics of the groin

Left outer aspect   Right outer aspect

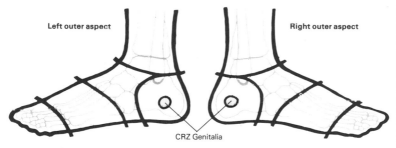

CRZ Genitalia

Sixth patient with Headache
Causal Relationships:
Respiratory tract infection
Symptoms occur in:
Zones of the Head
CRZ: Nose and throat; Lymphatics of the head and neck; Bronchi; Lungs;
Sinuses; Spleen (as in all infections);
Pelvic organs (Bladder, Genitalia) because of their reflex relationship to
the nose and throat; Liver and Kidneys (to aid elimination of metabolites).

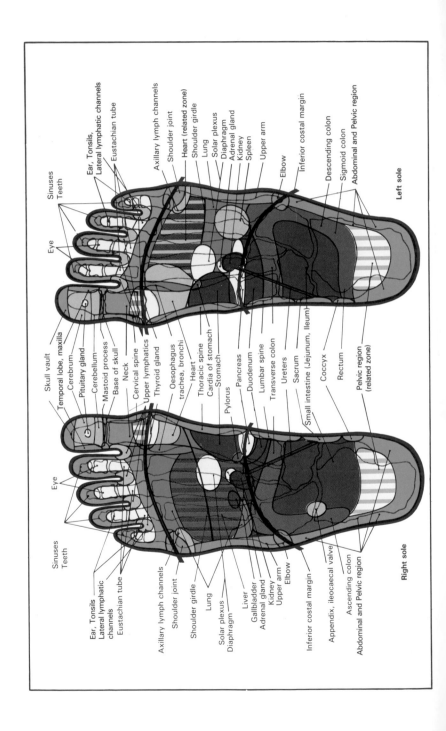

Left sole

Sinuses
Teeth

Eye

Ear, Tonsils,
Lateral lymphatic channels

Eustachian tube

Axillary lymph channels
Shoulder joint
Heart (related zone)
Shoulder girdle
Lung
Solar plexus
Diaphragm
Adrenal gland
Kidney
Spleen
Upper arm

Elbow

Inferior costal margin

Descending colon

Sigmoid colon

Abdominal and Pelvic region

Skull vault
Temporal lobe, maxilla
Cerebrum
Pituitary gland
Cerebellum
Mastoid process
Base of skull
Neck
Cervical spine
Upper lymphatics
Thyroid gland
Oesophagus
trachea, bronchi
Heart
Thoracic spine
Cardia of stomach
Stomach
Pylorus
Pancreas
Duodenum
Lumbar spine
Transverse colon
Ureters
Sacrum
Small intestine (Jejunum, Ileum)
Coccyx
Rectum
Pelvic region
(related zone)

Right sole

Sinuses
Teeth

Eye

Ear, Tonsils
Lateral lymphatic
channels
Eustachian tube

Axillary lymph channels
Shoulder joint
Shoulder girdle
Lung
Solar plexus
Diaphragm
Liver
Gallbladder
Adrenal gland
Kidney
Upper arm
Elbow

Inferior costal margin

Appendix, ileocaecal valve
Ascending colon
Abdominal and Pelvic region

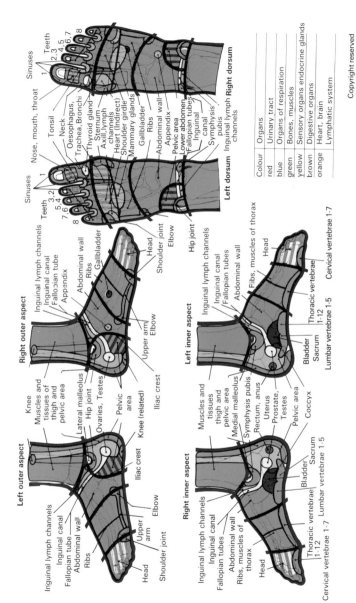

Left outer aspect

Inguinal lymph channels
Inguinal canal
Fallopian tube
Abdominal wall
Ribs
Upper arm
Elbow
Head
Shoulder joint
Iliac crest

Right outer aspect

Knee
Muscles and tissues of thigh and pelvic area
Lateral malleolus
Hip joint
Ovaries, Testes
Pelvic area
Knee (related)
Iliac crest
Inguinal lymph channels
Inguinal canal
Fallopian tube
Appendix
Abdominal wall
Ribs
Gallbladder
Head
Shoulder joint
Elbow
Upper arm
Elbow
Hip joint

Sinuses
Teeth
1
3, 2
5, 4
7, 6
8
Nose, mouth, throat
Tonsil
Neck
Oesophagus, Trachea, Bronchi
Thyroid gland
Sternum
Heart (indirect)
Axill.lymph channels
Shoulder girdle
Mammary glands
Gallbladder
Ribs
Abdominal wall
Appendix
Pelvic area
Lower abdomen
Fallopian tubes
Inguinal canal
Symphysis' pubis

Sinuses
Teeth
1
2, 3
4, 5
6, 7
8

Left dorsum   Inguinal lymph   **Right dorsum**
                   channels

Right inner aspect

Inguinal lymph channels
Inguinal canal
Fallopian tubes
Abdominal wall
Ribs, muscles of thorax
Head
Cervical vertebrae 1-7   Lumbar vertebrae 1-5
Thoracic vertebrae 1-12   Sacrum
Bladder
Coccyx
Pelvic area
Testes
Prostate,
Uterus
Symphysis pubis
Rectum, anus
Medial malleolus
Muscles and tissues thigh and pelvic area

Left inner aspect

Inguinal lymph channels
Inguinal canal
Fallopian tubes
Abdominal wall
Fibs, muscles of thorax
Head
Thoracic vertebrae 1-12
Sacrum
Bladder
Lumbar vertebrae 1-5
Cervical vertebrae 1-7

Colour	Organs
red	Urinary tract
blue	Organs of respiration
green	Bones, muscles
yellow	Sensory organs endocrine glands
brown	Digestive organs
orange	Heart, brain
	Lymphatic system

Diagram 19

This seventh patient presents you with a highly diverse treatment picture, because all the *single* disorders are combined now, and must have their relationships noted. This picture may easily change, and will also most certainly be enlarged by any additional findings at the first reflex zone massage, when it will be noted on general examination that the disturbed reflex zones react painfully, and that healthy ones do not.

Similarly, the entire disease picture of the individual with his respective wholly personal background will merge with the causal relationship. This therapy can direct one away from thinking of isolated symptoms and pathological concepts towards integrating all experience in one's concept of care.

Carefully graded treatment is valuable for both therapist and patient. The therapist will exercise her profession with greater commitment and devotion when she is engaged in a sensibly planned total regime, and is not just treating isolated parts of the patient at random.

Patients are, in many cases, already seeking healing and alleviation from unorthodox forms of medicine, and are not wholly dependent on the apparatus of modern medicine.

The merits of both forms can be assessed and recognized by anyone of sense, discernment and sensitivity. In any truly balanced organic therapy attempts should be made to restore an entire sense of well-being, including that of the psyche. One may extend this concept imaginatively by saying that a painful reflex zone to the gall-bladder gives, not only the impression of a physical state of illness, which may be confirmed in the laboratory, but also that in such a person 'the gall overflows'.

A painful reflex zone to the shoulder girdle gives, on the surface, evidence of tension in this area, but behind this there is frequently an additional psychical stress, so that the patient 'carries a heavy burden on his shoulders'. Another has an extremely sensitive zone to the intestine, suffers from flatulence and has little appetite, despite careful selection of diet, all of which indicate an organic problem. Such symptoms frequently disappear spontaneously when the patient is better able to 'digest' his problems,

An understanding of the relationship between body and mind is indeed well known. However, one must *remind oneself* daily and with each treatment in order that this vital link remains in the forefront of one's thinking and understanding. Reflex zone massage of the feet is a useful and effective form of treatment, making great demands on the therapist and on the patient. Because of this it can develop widely and has great possibilities for benefiting the sick.

It must be said that many diseases can be treated but not all people, since some lack the necessary will to be restored to health and well-being. There are also, sadly, those in whom the disease process or trauma has overwhelmed the body, and who cannot be restored to full health.

The task of an aspiring practitioner extends far beyond learning and applying the actual 'technique' of the grip-sequence. With skilled, imaginative and informed reflex zone massage to the feet the whole person can be treated. The therapist acquires a broad view of medicine and learns to apply her skills with compassion. She can also help the patient to assume responsibility for a healthier lifestyle.

SECTION II

22.
CASE HISTORIES

This section of the book has been put together from the written and verbal accounts of participants at the courses of instruction which I have given. Their actual practice has resulted in a wealth of material from which to choose, and the selection has been made with the aim of showing the diversity of conditions which have responded to reflex zone massage of the feet, supplemented by some from my own practice and experience.

The experiences and progress during treatment described on the pages which follow will never be exactly reproduced in another person with similar symptoms. Each person will react individually and differently.

One of the basic principles of reflex zone massage to the feet is reiterated here: It is not the illness which is treated, but the entire sick person.

ABDOMINAL CRAMPS

A housewife, aged 33, had suffered for a long time from abdominal cramps which she found unbearable. Beside the painful reflex zones to the entire digestive tract which were found on palpation, she had a wart 0.5cm thick on the right sole over the area of the small intestine.

She experienced some relief of her symptoms after the second reflex zone massage to the feet. The wart became visibly smaller with each successive treatment and the cramps were less painful. By the time she had had seven massages her bowel movements had returned to normal, she had less flatulence, and the pain had completely ceased. After twelve treatments, circulation of the skin to the area where the wart had formed was normal, and a year later she reported that she continued to feel well.

ACUTE EARACHE

When two-year-old Michael was brought by his mother for treatment he was crying and in obvious pain, rubbing his right ear with his fist. The ear was red and inflamed, but a closer inspection was not possible since he was in too much pain.

A firm hold was maintained on the reflex zone to the right ear for two minutes (using the sedation grip), and the child went to sleep in his mother's arms. He has had no recurrence of his earache.

ALLERGY

A shop assistant, 35 years old, suffered from repeated allergic rashes, which were at times accompanied by impaired consciousness. With each attack she had to spend several days in hospital. By chance, a therapist trained in reflex zone massage of the feet, and who had had a similar experience, was present on one of these occasions and examined her feet.

The reflex zones to the lymphatics, the endocrine glands, the liver and the spleen were extremely sensitive. Fifteen minutes after the initial examination and treatment, the rash, itching and lapses in consciousness became less marked, and the patient fell into a deep and refreshing sleep. A further eight treatments followed at intervals of three to four days, after which the reflex zones were relatively painless, and the allergy did not reappear.

ATAXIA

A six-year-old child with Rhesus negative blood suffered from ataxia and an almost unintelligible pronunciation due to excessive salivation. It had been stated that she would have to enter a special school, although she was not mentally handicapped.

On palpation, all the reflex zones to the head were taut and tense, and those to the thyroid gland, urogenital tract, and the lymphatics of the throat and pelvis were very sensitive to touch. After the second treatment the hands of the child were noticeably more still, salivation started to diminish, and her speech and ataxia started to improve.

She had fifteen treatments in two months, and subsequently passed the entrance test to the local elementary school. Reflex zone massages to the feet were continued at longer intervals, as she was still apt to salivate excessively when under stress. Only a few further treatments were necessary as time went on, and her ataxia disappeared completely.

BACKACHE
A sixty-year-old housewife lay stiffly in bed, and had been unable to get up for three days because of acute pain in her right leg and over the coccyx.

The first reflex zone massage to the feet was carried out very lightly and, because she was in such pain, it was conducted in the same rhythm as her breathing. Treatment was concentrated in the reflex zones of the lower spine and the pelvic organs on the right side. After fifteen minutes the pain lessened perceptibly. The patient was anxious about trying to move at all, but was persuaded to try and move her right leg, to find that there was no limitation of movement in either her right leg or her back. She tried walking to the dining room and back, and soon fell asleep, considerably relieved and relaxed. The next morning, her urine, which had been left standing undisturbed for some time, was found to contain a heavy reddish sediment. The day after that she was able to resume her normal household activities unaided.

BED-WETTING
An eight-year-old child wet the bed every night. There was a distinct visible swelling over the bladder zone on the feet, which was also painful when touched. It was found on physical examination that the reflex zones to the head were even more painful when touched than were those of the pelvic areas. After the child had had four treatments, the family moved to another town, but reported eight months later that the child had not wet his bed again after receiving the second treatment.

BILIARY COLIC
The following account was given by a masseur: During the course of a severe infection, a patient suffered a sudden attack of biliary colic, of which there had been no warning. The reflex zone therapist who was summoned applied firm pressure on both dorsal and plantar aspects of the foot to the reflex zone to the gall-bladder, and after about ten seconds the pain was relieved. The patient suffered no side effects from this treatment.

BRONCHITIS
A five-year-old girl had suffered from bronchitis since infancy. Most of the time she breathed with her mouth open, and her sinuses were troublesome. Her sleep was disturbed, and she had no appetite.

The reflex zones of the feet were treated with great care, since the child would cry at the slightest touch. After the second treatment she slept uninterruptedly through the night, and was noticeably more cheerful and communicative in the morning. For no apparent reason she developed a runny nose, which stopped after five days, but there was no other sign of a cold. She was now able to bear more pressure on the reflex zones. Her pale, crying manner gradually gave way to an impression of health and rosiness. Ten weeks later she had a medical examination, at which it was found that her nasal polyps had disappeared, and that her tonsils were no longer enlarged and inflamed.

BUERGER'S DISEASE

A 67-year-old engineer, who smoked forty cigarettes daily, was unable to walk for a distance of more than fifty metres without having to take a long rest. Before the therapist agreed to start a course of reflex zone massage to the feet, he was asked to stop smoking completely, which he agreed to do.

Initially, all the reflex zones of the feet were painful on palpation. It was only after eight treatments that the pain began to be concentrated in the reflex zones to the respiratory tract, the heart and the pelvic organs. From the second treatment onward he began to produce copious amounts of unusually coloured sputum, and this persisted undiminished for six weeks. After he had had sixteen treatments the patient was able to walk for up to three hours without pain and without having to stop for a rest.

CERVICAL SYNDROME

About ten years previously a 57-year-old housewife had needed an upper denture. For eight years she had suffered from increasing disability in the cervical spine. X-rays revealed no abnormality, and she did not respond to any tablets, injections, or the heat treatment which had been recommended.

The first reflex zone massage of the feet resulted in a sharp piercing pain in the reflex zone to the rear molar teeth on the left. After two intensive treatments the left side of the woman's face became extremely painful, red and swollen. X-rays of the jaw showed that a large piece of the root of the tooth was still present, which required surgery for its removal. Following the extraction the patient suffered no further pain or disability in her neck or cervical spine.

CHRONIC CONSTIPATION

A 71-year-old woman, who was thin and haggard-looking, had been having mudpacks applied in an attempt to relieve the pain she felt in her hip, but with no effect. On questioning, it was found that she had for some years suffered from an intestinal complaint.

Findings: The tissues of both feet were atonic, and presented a wrinkled and 'worn' appearance. The reflex zones to all her joints and to the alimentary tract were sensitive. She commenced having reflex zone massage of the feet, and after five treatments the pain in her hip lessened, but her irregular bowel habits persisted. However, the skin of her feet began to improve from one treatment to another, regaining some elasticity while the tissues recovered some tone. The white coat on her tongue began to disappear. At this time she began to break out into nightly sweats, which had a strong odour, and for some days she had a rash of pimples all over her skin. From the eleventh treatment onward her bowel habits became more regular, although she had a lot of flatulence which had an offensive smell, and her stools were hard and dark brown.

After thirty treatments her bowel habits had become quite normal, and she presented an altogether fresher and livelier appearance.

CIRCULATORY DISTURBANCE FOLLOWING THE INSERTION OF HIP PROSTHESES

A 75-year-old patient had had two hip prostheses (artificial hip joints) inserted within a period of eighteen months. He complained of severe circulatory disturbance in the veins of the right calf, and pain and limitation of movement in the leg.

He was sceptical and anxious at the beginning of the treatment course, fearing that reflex zone massage to the feet might worsen his condition. Cautious examination of the feet revealed that reflex zones to all the joints and the spine were painful, and that the reflex zone to the left kidney could hardly be touched. The results of the first treatment were encouraging, as his legs felt warm and relaxed that whole night. However, the patient had to pass urine six times during the night. After only a few massages he was able to take longer walks, and found that walking on hard pavements did not worry him, as it had previously. After six weeks he was able to take his first walk up a mountain incline, to his great delight.

CIRCULATORY DISTURBANCE IN THE HEAD

A 54-year-old sales representative had been receiving medical treatment for many years for a circulatory disorder. He had had several thromboses. Since the summer of 1972, his most disturbing symptoms had been headaches, fainting fits, and more recently he had been having attacks of weakness, and was no longer able to work. Whilst in hospital he had had an EEG, which showed evidence of some abnormality in the left upper cerebrum, but it was uncertain whether this was due to early cerebral haemorrhage or a brain tumour.

The first reflex zone massage to the feet had to be carried out with extreme care, since all the reflex zones were very painful. After the third treatment the sensation of pressure in his head was alleviated, and the painful reflex zones were concentrated in those to the head, heart and pelvic areas. With continuing treatment the intervals between his attacks grew longer. An EEG was repeated three months later, and was normal, Since then the patient has been free of all his complaints.

In some astonishment the patient remarked that his toes were also now quite free from pain, and that for the first time in thirty years he did not have to have special shoes made for him to accommodate his previously painful toes.

CONSTIPATION AND CRYING FITS IN A CHILD

A child who was 5½-years-old would only sleep in a lighted room, woke frequently during the night, and would cry for hours on end without anyone knowing why he was so distressed. He was reserved in nature, and found it difficult to communicate or play with other children, and unless he was given laxatives he had no bowel action.

Findings: The big toe was markedly swollen on the plantar surface. There were painful reflex zones to the solar plexus and the ascending colon.

He came for reflex zone massage to the feet twice a week. After he had had ten treatments he had changed into a playful youngster, was able to sleep at night without needing the light on, and had a normal bowel action daily. No further laxatives were needed.

CONVULSIONS IN AN INFANT

When she was about six months old, X, a twin, suffered from her first attack of convulsions. She was investigated extensively in a

Neurological Clinic, but her condition did not improve. The infant lay limply and listlessly on her back, and any attempts to sit her up failed.

Findings: Both feet were icy cold, particularly the toes, and the pads on the soles of the big toes were taut and swollen. On the dorsum of the feet over the metatarso-phalangeal joints was a firm and swollen area which was very sensitive to touch. After the first three treatments had been very carefully carried out, the mother said that she felt there was some improvement, in that the child seemed to be trying to respond to the parents attempts to communicate with her. After the fourth treatment she was able to hold a sitting position for a short while, and did not immediately collapse. While she was in a sitting position it was noticed that the left half of the thoracic cage was underdeveloped.

The feet became perceptibly warmer with each treatment, and she started to move them about more. She also began to make efforts to crawl. After twelve treatments it was possible to communicate almost normally with X. However, the left side of the thoracic cage continued to sag.

Three months elapsed before she was given a further course of reflex zone massage to the feet, as she now tended to fall to one side when trying to walk. There had, in the meantime, been a great improvement in the condition of the reflex zones of her feet, and the only ones which were found to be marginally abnormal were those of the head and lower spine, which improved after a further eight treatments. Her walking became normal, and she is now indistinguishable from her twin.

DISTURBANCE OF TASTE

The 43-year-old wife of a wine-grower came for treatment as she had osteochondrosis. Disconsolately she recounted that for the past eight months all that she had eaten and drunk had tasted of vinegar. Treatment by a variety of specialists had brought about no improvement.

Palpation of the feet revealed painful zones to the head, neck, lymphatics and upper abdomen. After the third treatment she noticed that from time to time she had a different perception of taste. After ten treatments she arrived to say that she had eaten six pieces of birthday cake to celebrate having recovered her sense of taste, and she said 'that it tasted even better than it had before'. A total of sixteen treatments was given and her condition did not recur.

DEPRESSION

A 50-year-old manager had suffered from acute depression for eighteen months, and was heavily sedated with tranquillizers and sleeping tablets. His General Practitioner had said that if his depression continued she recommended that he see a psychiatrist. The depression felt like a physical burden to him, and he could hardly bear to get out of bed in the morning. He had lost all interest in life, ceased to go out, and was just trying to get through each day at work mechanically. He had considered suicide, and was retaining the option.

The first examination and palpation were short, as he hated to be touched, and only head zones, which were exquisitely tender, were palpated. However, he said that he had slept well that night when he came again for treatment, and this time a complete palpation of all the reflex zones was carried out. Those of the kidneys, adrenals, head, neck, solar plexus, pylorus and ileo-caecal valve were all very tender.

After the second treatment he noticed that his urinary output increased, and experienced the same sense of relaxation after treatment. He came twice a week for treatment, and after the fourth was able to dispense with his sleeping tablets. He then started to sweat profusely, which lasted for four days, but as he was sleeping well and feeling less heavily weighed down by a sense of physical oppression this did not worry him. After six treatments his salivation increased for 48 hours, and after eight treatments he found that his eyes filled with tears several times during that week, though he had not cried for many years.

After fourteen treatments he had stopped taking all drugs, had started to go out again with his friends, and realized to his delight that he was singing at the weekends. He still has occasional feelings of depression, but feels more able to take time off to allow them to pass naturally, otherwise he takes an active an alert interest in the world around him, and feels an occasional sense of *joie de vivre*, which he says he had completely forgotten. He no longer feels a sense of distaste at being touched, and has made efforts to improve his posture, standing more erectly and allowing his shoulders to drop rather than being hunched up round his ears.

DYSMENORRHOEA

A 38-year-old woman complained of severe pain preceding and during her menstrual periods. The cycles were irregular, and were accompanied by depression.

Her feet were visibly grey, and the tissues were atonic. There were callosities over the thyroid and diaphragmatic reflex zones, and there was a hard, horny area of skin about 6mm thick on each heel (over the reflex zones to the pelvic organs). There was a brown liver spot about the size of a pea over the reflex zone to the sacrum.

The feet were cool to the touch, and were in general painful when handled with light pressure. The first two treatments only lasted for ten minutes as the patient very quickly showed signs of overdosage. On the third visit she arrived feeling surprisingly well, and informed me that she had been sleeping well, soundly and dreamlessly. The foot was now normal to touch, and the pain which she had felt to be unbearable during massage of the reflex zones to the pelvic organs and endocrine system had diminished somewhat.

After the sixth treatment she began to menstruate. Her period was not accompanied by any of the symptoms which had troubled her previously, and there was no swelling or feeling of tension in her breasts. During her period the patient was given a light and gentle massage to the reflex zones of the genitalia, and after menstruation had ceased she suffered a malodorous vaginal discharge, which persisted until the next ovulation. After this she felt better than she had for a long while, but was advised to take regular Sitz baths to completely stabilize her condition.

EAR INFECTION

When he was eighteen years old a masseur of 37 had developed pyelonephritis and haematuria. He had also suffered from angina when he was young. For the past six months he had been having sensations of pressure and tension in both ears, which were almost painful. He was found on medical examination to have cochlear degeneration, which it was said might have been caused by environmental factors such as noise, exhaust fumes, or something similar. The damage was considered to be irreparable, likely to worsen with age, and no form of therapy was thought likely to be effective, and none had therefore been recommended.

Palpation of the feet showed painful reflex zones to the tonsils, upper lymphatics, both kidneys and the pelvic organs. After the first treatment the symptoms in his ears disappeared spontaneously, and they have not recurred.

FACIAL NEURALGIA

A 45-year-old housewife came for theapy as she had been suffering from facial neuralgia for many years.

Painful reflex zones to the sinuses, the left ear and the bronchi were found on the feet. Between the fourth and fifth toes on the left she had athlete's foot, which she was treating with local applications of an antimycotic product. Every time she stopped treatment the infection recurred a few days later. The first three treatments resulted only in her feeling a sense of general relaxation and sleeping more deeply. After the fourth treatment a pyrexial, flu-like illness developed abruptly, with almost purulent mucus secretions from the nose and throat. The patient had never before experienced such a violent illness. On the advice of her doctor she allowed the fever to run its course naturally without taking any anti-pyrexial drugs. When she recovered she was no longer troubled with neuralgia, and the athlete's foot healed spontaneously shortly thereafter.

FROZEN SHOULDER

A farmer, who was 61 years of age, had suffered from a 'frozen shoulder' for eighteen months. A variety of treatments, injections, and thirty massages to the affected area combined with hot mudpacks had brought him no relief.

There was a conspicuous hallux valgus on both feet. The reflex zones to the spine, the shoulder girdle, the liver and both kidneys were sensitive to pressure.

He began to be able to move his shoulder more freely after four treatments. He then suffered an offensive diarrhoea for 24 hours. After fifteen treatments his symptoms disappeared completely, and today, three years later, he is able to carry out all the work on his farm without limitation of movement of the shoulder or arm.

GASTRITIS

A lawyer, aged 49 years, had suffered for many years from gastritis, which was accompanied by heartburn and attacks of acidic belching. From an examination of the feet it was seen that the reflex zones to the upper abdomen, the small intestine, the rectum and anus were sensitive. A scar was discovered at the reflex zone to the pylorus, and the patient had no memory of an event which could have given rise to such a scar.

The scar was treated by an injection of procaine (Huneke's

neural therapy), and soon after this the patient experienced a feeling of warmth and relaxation over the whole of the upper abdomen. As the patient's symptoms disappeared completely after this treatment, and he was kept busy at his office, it was a year before he came for another treatment, this time for an injury which he had sustained at sports practice. There had been no recurrence of his abdominal discomfort during this year.

HAEMORRHOIDS

An office worker, 53 years old, had for months been using suppositories and ointments in an attempt to relieve her itching and bleeding piles. Before undergoing surgery, she wanted to try reflex zone massage to the feet to see whether it offered her any relief.

On visual examination the zones around the inner malleoli (which correspond to the reflex zones of the true pelvis) were taut, swollen, and the skin was friable and blue/grey in colour. On palpation the reflex zones to the small and large intestine and the base of the spine were distinctly abnormal. During the first four massages the taut area over the ankles was not touched, as the woman was naturally worried about the possibility of infection here. In place of this, the corresponding reflex zones in the wrists were massaged thoroughly, after which the dark discolouration and swelling around the ankles noticeably subsided, and these areas could subsequently be included in the treatment of the feet.

The nightly itch eased, and her bowels were opened without pain or blood loss. After a series of twenty treatments the patient again visited her doctor, who decided that surgery was now not necessary. The patient noticed and commented on the fact that her thighs and buttocks were no longer cold, and that she was able to walk more easily.

HEADACHE

An eleven-year-old girl had suffered from left-sided headache since her younger sister had been born when she was five years old. Initially these headaches had occured every six to eight weeks, but she was now having them every ten days.

Findings: On the feet the reflex zones to the left side of the head were abnormal, and those of the urinary system, the lumbo-sacral spine and the genital tract were also painful. After the third reflex zone massage of the feet her headaches became less intense, and after the seventh massage it was seen that her cheeks were rosier. There followed a long interval in the treatment sessions as the family were away on holiday. During this time she had a vague feeling of being unwell at about three weekly intervals. After some months she had a further six treatments and for the last two years she has been a normal, healthy child.

HEART AILMENT

An engineer of 55 years old had received reflex zone massage of the feet at various times in the past. As well as backache, he now complained of a deterioration of the heart condition from which he had suffered for the past eight years, and which had not improved through the administration of any of the drugs which he had been given. He had symptoms of ataxia, and said that he felt anxious and uncertain whilst driving his car.

Physical examination of the feet showed negligible abnormality of the reflex zone to the heart. The reflex zones of the liver, gall-bladder, diaphragm, stomach, small intestine and shoulder girdle were more sensitive to pressure. The first treatment resulted in a release of tension in the musculature of the back and shoulder girdle, and the patient stated that he felt able to breathe more easily. During a series of ten treatments he suffered from excessive flatulence, but his bowel action returned to normal. He was advised to take a sauna bath once a week, which he does, and for the last two years he has been free of all symptoms.

HICCUPS

An office worker of 52 years of age who was considerably overworked developed hiccups, which persisted for six hours. When the office closed he came for treatment, feeling very depressed. Constant, light pressure for two minutes to the reflex zone of the diaphragm was sufficient to stop the hiccups.

HYDROCEPHALUS

A fifteen-month-old infant was brought from a local nursing home for treatment. When she was not sleeping, eating or crying, she lay apathetically in her cot. She was unable to sit, stand up or walk, and she did not talk. When she was awake she moved her head from side to side in a continuous rocking movement. As soon as her head stopped moving she would cry out. Medical opinion stated that she was an idiot.

Findings: The big toes were swollen, taut and tense. After the first reflex zone massage to the feet she spontaneously stopped rocking her head from side to side, and she seemed to be calmer. After the second treatment, to the astonishment of the mother and the therapist, she pulled herself into a sitting position with great effort. She attempted to stand after the third treatment. From the seventh treatment onward she behaved in a normal fashion for her age.

When treatment was started on this child her head circumference was 46.5 cm. This remained the same while she grew in body length from 62 cm to 74 cm, by which time the relationship between the circumference of the head and the body length was evidently normal.

After two years — the child is now little more than three years old — the impression that she gave was that of being a normal toddler. Her physical development is retarded by about four months, and arrangements have been made for her to have a further series of reflex zone massages to her feet.

HYPERTENSION

A 58-year-old textile merchant was 30 kg overweight, and complained of sensations of pressure in his head, fainting, restless sleep, nervousness, and said that he had little appetite for food. His blood pressure was 195/95.

On examination, the tissues of his feet were generally rough and grey, and the reflex zones of the upper abdomen and head were very sensitive to touch. He was considerably distressed by the pain which he experienced during the first treatment, and wanted time to consider whether or not he would return for a second treatment. He returned three days later in some dudgeon, as he had been considerably troubled by diarrhoea and flatulence during that time. In the meantime, the reflex zones had become a little less painful. His treatment continued, and after the fifth reflex zone massage to the feet the man came to terms with this unusual method of treatment. He told friends and acquaintances that his symptoms had been relieved, and that he now felt very well.

He allowed himself to be persuaded that his sumptuous evening meals were harming rather than helping him, and managed to lose 20 kg in four months. Eighteen months later he had a medical examination, at which it was found that his blood pressure and liver function test had returned to normal.

HYPERTHYROIDISM

A 39-year-old businesswoman, the mother of four lively children, complained of increasing hyperthyroidism. She was losing weight rapidly, cried at the least provocation, and could not sleep at night.

The first reflex zone massage of the feet was concluded after ten minutes, since the patient began to cry violently and was beginning to shiver. A thorough palpation of the reflex zones was only possible at the second treatment, and was carried out lightly and delicately. This showed abnormal reflex zones to the entire endocrine system, as well as to the solar plexus and head.

The following treatments consisted predominantly of soothing, stroking movements. From the fifth treatment her condition began to stabilize, and she became less agitated. After the eighth treatment she menstruated normally, without pain and with relatively little blood loss. Shortly afterwards the feeling that she had previously had of having a lump in her throat began to disappear along with her dysphagia. She had gained 16 kg in weight after sixteen treatments, and said that she felt as though she was once more in control of her life.

HYPOTENSION

A businesswoman, aged 34, slightly built and anxious, with a blood pressure of 90/65, came for treatment. She explained that she did not feel that there was anything 'organically' wrong, but said that she felt like ' a wilting house plant'.

Findings: All the reflex zones from the heel to the toes were painful for the first three massages. At the beginning of the fourth treatment the patient burst into tears, and was encouraged to cry freely. This release of tension was evident on the feet immediately thereafter when the reflex zone to the solar plexus (which is the same as that to the diaphragm) was no longer painful, and neither was there, to the astonishment of both patient and practitioner, much pain in any of the other reflex zones. After fourteen treatments her condition had improved so much that she was able to resume work feeling restored. Her blood pressure stabilized at 120/90, and her sleep became deep and restful.

IMPAIRED VISION

An active, alert, retired woman of 72 years of age, had suffered severe impairment of her vision over the past three months, for no apparent cause. Since she did not wish to go into an old people's home, she had tried every available means of treatment to restore her sight, but had not been helped by any of them. She decided that she would try a course of reflex zone massage to the feet as a last resort.

On palpation the reflex zones to the eyes, kidneys and bladder were very painful. Between the second and third toes she had athlete's foot, which was very irritating, had persisted for four months, and for which she had no explanation as to its cause.

After the second treatment the patient began to sleep more soundly at night, and did not have to get up to empty her bladder two to four times during the night as had previously been the case.

At the third treatment she said that the dark veil which had lain in front of her eyes had lightened, and that she was now able to distinguish colours again. After the fourth treatment she was able to read her Bible. Over the next four years she came for a further four series of treatments, none of which were for her poor sight, but because she had some other ailments which commonly occur in old age.

INFECTED FOCUS IN A TOOTH

A professional sportsman, aged 21, had had severe pain in the lumbo-sacral spine for several weeks. Various methods of treatment were tried, but brought him no relief. He was not able to participate in any sporting activity unless he had previously been given pain-killing injections.

The reflex zones to the lower half of the spine were very sensitive on palpation, and so, surprisingly, were the reflex zones to the head. After the third treatment he developed a temperature and a very severe toothache. The dentist found an infected focus in his apparently healthy teeth, after the extraction of which his backache disappeared.

INFECTIOUS HEPATITIS

This account of her own illness was sent in by a therapist: "One year ago I became acutely ill with viral hepatitis. For weeks beforehand I had noticed that there was pain over the areas of my feet which represented the liver, stomach and solar plexus while standing, but which became concentrated in one small area in the reflex zone of the liver until the outbreak of the illness. A sharply defined bluish area of about 1 cm in diameter was also plainly visible over this point.

During my stay in hospital I frequently worked on the sensitive reflex zones of the upper abdomen and spleen. I could hardly touch the reflex zone to the liver. As my condition improved the reflex zone to the liver became less painful to palpation, and the bluish point disappeared, but remains today, barely visible, as a pale yellow discolouration of the skin.''

INTERMITTENT CLAUDICATION

A 48-year-old industrial consultant came for treatment, and was found to have greatly swollen legs, in which he complained of severe cramp-like pains. His hearing, vision and memory had deteriorated, and he complained of circulatory problems and backache as well. There were hard callouses on both heels around the area corresponding to the pelvic organs and at the base of the toe joints, corresponding to the neck region. Palpation verified visual observation, as all the reflex zones to the pelvis, the head and the shoulder girdle were sensitive. Results showed themselves after the first treatment by reflex zone massage of the feet in a relaxation of tension in the entire musculature of the back and legs.

This man required fifteen treatments before he was once more without pain and able to return to work. The nightly pacing about his room with cramps in the legs and tension and excessive warmth of the feet ceased as the pain was relieved, and he was visibly restored to health.

IRRITABLE BLADDER

A lively and busy seamstress of 50 years of age had suffered from an irritable bladder for the past three years. No organic disorder was found on gynaecological or urological examination. On the feet the reflex zones to the bladder, the solar plexus, the lumbo-sacral spine and, more than any other, the reflex zone to the pharynx, were painful. After the first treatment she found that she only needed to empty her bladder every three hours, but she developed a heavy cold which lasted for two days and then disappeared.

Six reflex zone massages to the feet were all that were needed by this patient before she was relieved of all her symptoms. A year later she remains well.

KIDNEY STONES

A mechanical engineer, 54 years old, had had a kidney stone

removed previously by means of a basket procedure. When he was discovered to have a stone forming in his kidney two years later he decided to try a series of reflex zone massages to the feet before undergoing further surgery.

The findings were of strong pain in the reflex zones to the left kidney and the lower spine. After two intensive treatments the patient stated that the nature of the pain had changed, in that it was now lower down and tracking further downwards towards his bladder. He deduced that the stone was descending down the ureter. After eleven days, two stones entered the bladder, and he had colicky pain and haematuria. Two days later the stones were passed in the urine, and were found on examination to be oxalate stones.

MIGRAINE

A 42-year-old patient complained of almost daily attacks of migraine headache, which he had been having with increasing severity for the past ten years. Because of his frequent absences from work, he was about to lose his position.

On palpation the reflex zones of the head, liver, stomach and lymphatic system were sensitive. The feet were treated at intervals of three days. After the seventh treatment the man was no longer in need of the usual drugs for his headaches, and his headaches did not recur even at times of great stress at work. He was given, in all, fourteen massages to the reflex zones of the feet, and noted with some astonishment that his circulation had greatly improved, even though he was no longer taking any drugs for this either.

OSTEOARTHRITIS

An hotelier of 68 years of age came for treatment because of severe pain in all her large joints. She was hardly capable of dressing and undressing herself, and had tried several other remedies, but gained no relief from them.

Examination of the feet showed that the reflex zones to the kidneys and the entire alimentary tract were more sensitve to touch than were those of the large joints. After five treatments the reactions took the form of her passing frequent and foetid stools and urine, but her joints were becoming more free in their movement. She was given twelve treatments in all, and reported a year later that she had remained well. The following autumn she returned for two prophylactic treatments.

PARALYTIC ILEUS

Post-operative report: Following surgery for removal of a kidney stone, the patient developed a paralytic ileus. Enemas and other convential treatments did not bring about any improvement, and the condition of the patient worsened rapidly.

Reflex zone massage to the feet was carried out by a doctor friend who was, by chance, visiting the patient at that time. Within a very few minutes of treatment some bowel sounds were heard. The prompt effectiveness of this treatment reminded both the doctor and the patient of the 'seconds phenomenon' described by Huneke.

PERIPHERONEUROPATHY IN A PATIENT WITH DIABETES MELLITUS

A 48-year-old engineer had severe cramps in his legs three or four nights a week and suffered from diabetes mellitus, for which he took forty units of Lente insulin daily. He had mature onset diabetes at the age of forty, had had two cataract operations, and was, as is usual prone to many infections.

At the first visit, all the reflex zones were painful, but particularly the reflex zones of the stomach, pancreas, head, kidneys and adrenals and those of the spine. Treatment was carried out gently and he was asked to check his urine carefully at each voiding. After the first treatment he felt somewhat relaxed, but suffered from mild hypoglycaemia the following day. He was only able to come for treatment once a week because he had to travel some distance. After the second treatment he experienced some diminution in the intensity of the cramps, and noted that his glycosuria was down from two to nought for 24 to 48 hours after treatment, and that he felt 'light-headed' for two days after treatment. His urinary output increased, and was followed by first an increase in the bronchial secretions and then of stools. These were not very marked except for the 48 hours after each treatment.

After six treatments he asked if it was possible that therapy could influence his insulin requirement, for he was eating more and had reduced his insulin to 36 units per day. He admitted that he had always been hungry on the strict diet he had kept to beforehand, and now felt satisfied after each meal. The cramps in his legs were now very infrequent, perhaps one a week or not at all and he was drinking the bottle of tonic water that he had been asked to take each day.

After twenty treatments his insulin requirement was down to 22 units of Lente insulin daily, he had had no cramps for several weeks, and his resistance to minor infections had increased. He also said that he had noticed an improvement in proprioception.

This man's condition has remained stable for the past two years, with no recurrence of the cramps in his leg. He comes for treatment two or three times a year if he feels he is developing a cold or an infection, or because an old injury to his back flares up whenever he has to lift anything heavy. Three or four treatments usually suffice before he is well again. The reflex zones to the eyes and the pancreas remain more sensitive to palpation than do any others.

PROSTATITIS WITH MICTURITION DIFFICULTIES
A participant at one of the courses learned from the partner with whom he was working that the reflex zone to the prostate gland was particularly sensitive. At that time he was not aware of any symptoms. Eight weeks later he developed painful prostatitis and had difficulty in passing urine. On rectal examination the prostate gland was found to be hypertrophied.

The symptoms were alleviated after ten reflex zone massages to his feet. He no longer had frequency during the night and his urinary stream was strong. A medical examination confirmed that the prostate gland was normal.

PYLORIC STENOSIS
A four-month-old boy, the only child of friends, was due to have surgery in two weeks time for pyloric stenosis. A reflex zone therapist asked if she could see the feet of the baby.

She found on palpation that there was a painful response on the precise area of the reflex zone to the stomach and solar plexus. The next day she was told that, for the first time, the infant had taken his feed without vomiting afterwards. He was given a further two treatments, and his grandmother was shown how to massage the sensitive zones carefully, and asked to do so each evening.

Six months later the baby was again brought on a visit. As his condition had improved so markedly, it had not been necessary for him to have the operation which had been planned.

PYREXIAL INFECTION
A quiet, thin, sensitive child of seven had suffered for more than

a year from chronic sniffles, a feeling of heaviness in his head, general lassitude and pyrexial infections. He had to be protected from inclement weather, otherwise it was found that he would sustain a fever the following day and have to be put to bed. He was not making any progress at school.

Examination of the feet showed the reflex zones to the bronchi, sinuses, kidneys and spleen to be very painful. After the third and fourth treatments, the previously watery catarrh from which he had suffered became yolk-coloured, and he developed a slight cough. Following the sixth reflex zone massage to the feet, the boy reported with amazement that he was able to smell things again, and that the sense of pressure in his head was not so great.

He had, in all, ten treatments, each given quite precisely up to the level of his pain threshold. When he was caught in the rain one day he suffered no relapse, and eighteen months later the boy gives the impression of being bright and lively.

RECTAL PROLAPSE

An 83-year-old woman had suffered from a rectal prolapse since the birth of her last child.

Examination of the feet revealed that all the reflex zones to the entire pelvic area were abnormal. After the first treatment she no longer experienced a sensation of pressure round the anus, and a further four treatments confirmed this spontaneous resolution of her ailment.

SCIATICA

A carpenter, aged 46, had not been able to work for six weeks because of sciatica. Heat treatments, injections and salves had brought him no relief. He came limping and in obvious pain for treatment.

The reflex zones of the true pelvis, the lower spine, and particularly those of the kidneys were very painful when touched. This seemed strange, as the man said his urine was clear and micturition caused him no problems. After the first reflex zone massage he was able to walk a little more easily, and after the third treatment he was free of pain when walking. After four treatments he was able to return to work. However, his urine was now dark and cloudy, and gave off a strong odour. After eight treatments his urine returned to normal in colour, volume and odour, and the pain finally disappeared completely, both while walking and at rest.

TOOTH EXTRACTION

A 37-year-old saleswoman had a tooth extracted from her upper jaw. As a result, a sinus had formed between the maxilla and the nose. When breathing in she was aware of a passage of air from the mouth to the nose through this sinus. She had been told by the dentist that it would heal in time without surgery.

She was given ten treatments to the reflex zones of the feet to see what effect they had. At the end of this course of treatment the sinus had healed completely and she was free of pain and discomfort.

TORTICOLLIS (Wryneck)

Overnight a 55-year-old car salesman developed an extremely painful and stiff neck. It was only with great difficulty that he was able to move his head, neck or shoulder girdle.

He was given reflex zone massage to the feet for ten minute periods at a time in his home. This consisted largely of a careful but sustained rotation of the basal joint of the big toe, which brought about a reflex relaxation of the musculature of the neck. The immobility and acute pain resolved spontaneously and there was no recurrence of it. That evening he was able to sell three cars!

TREATMENT FOLLOWING A FALL FROM A HORSE

A manufacturer of 39, who was a passionate rider, fell from his horse, and suffered extensive bruising over the upper part of his spine and left shoulder. He was taken by a friend to hospital where several X-rays were taken, which showed that no fractures had been sustained, and then brought for reflex zone massage to the feet. The pain was relieved within thirty minutes, and the man was able to walk away unaided after the treatment was over. He was given a further three massages to promote healing of the bruised tissues.

UNDESCENDED TESTES

A twelve-year-old boy, whose teacher complained of his lack of concentration and his apathy, had not, so far, responded to any of the tonics prescribed for him. Physical examination of the feet showed disturbed circulation in the genital area, the head, the adrenal and the stomach reflex zones. A medical examination was made and he was diagnosed as having crypto-orchidism.

Over the course of ten reflex zone massages to the feet the

testes descended to a normal position. He subsequently found his schoolwork much easier to attend to, and a year later was one of the best pupils in the class.

VARICOSE VEINS

A 36-year-old waitress compained of marked congestion and pain in the veins of her legs. On the right shin there was a hot and somewhat reddened area. As there were, however, no varicose veins on her feet and ankles, palpation of the reflex zones of the feet was possible. The reflex zones to the pelvic organs, (particularly those of the rectum and anus), the liver, small intestine and spleen were very painful.

After the first treatment, the patient reported that she experienced 'lightening' of the pain in her legs for about six hours. The red area on the shin was treated by massaging the corresponding area on the forearm of the same side. Although very light pressure had been applied a haematoma developed on the forearm over this area, but the angry red area on the shin disappeared.

Over the course of fourteen reflex zone massages to the feet the bones of the ankles became visible once more as the ankles slimmed down, and the reflex zones of this area were no longer painful. The patient remarked that following the third treatment her urinary output had increased markedly, and that her menstrual irregularities were no longer evident.

SECTION III

23.

GENERAL PATTERNS OF TREATMENT

The following guidelines for treatment have been drawn up after many years of clinical practice and experience in reflex zone massage of the feet. They cannot be regarded as any more than an orientation to the general pattern that treatment should follow.

Far more important than the prescriptions printed here is the grasp and understanding of the complexity of the personal disease background of the individual, and the close observation of reactions in every single patient as soon as they occur.

This depends in *every case* on thorough, individual, visual and physical examination during the first reflex zone massage of the feet, from which a composite picture is developed. These observations form the guideline for the treatment which follows, but it must constantly be borne in mind that the reactions which manifest in the patient can bring about modification of the findings and consequent treatment pattern.

Visual observation provides you with the first indication of abnormal reflex zones on the feet. In order to have validity they must always be enhanced and verified by physical palpation.

Painful reflex zones arise because of disease which is still insignificant and not yet clinically detectable; because of weakness or overtaxation of an organ, or as the result of acute or chronic disorders. Reflex zones which are painful on the first reflex zone massage are divided into two groups:

(i) The symptomatic zones, in which treatment will be concentrated initially, and

(ii) The causal reflex zones, the discovery of which will illuminate the background to the presenting symptoms, accurately indicating those tissues, organs or systems which are under stress.

Causal reflex zones, (abbreviated as CRZ), are reflex zones which are either:

(a)   those in which the weakness or disability with which the patient presents originate, or

(b)   those which have been handicapped by the disease process, (e.g. the reflex zone to the solar plexus when pain is present, the reflex zones of the lymphatic system in infections), or both.

The following list of symptomatic and causal reflex zones must be tested in order to prove its aptness and veracity in each individual patient during the first reflex zone massage of the feet; and in order that your treatment departs from this static, prescribed form and brings to life a creative skilfulness. These guidelines for treatment will then be what they are intended to be: a sign post, which is not the pathway itself, but which points the direction.

Naturally, the schematic presentation of this mixed table cannot comprehend the individual variations on all feet. This comprehension can only be attained by constant, vigilant observation and sensitive palpation.

ALLERGY, ECZEMA
Symptomatic zones: Endocrine system, lymphatics.
CRZ: Liver and gall-bladder, small intestine, large intestine, kidneys, spleen, solar plexus; focus of infection; attention to diet!

APOPLEXY
Symptomatic zones: All the organs of the head (particularly the big toe, which is the site of cerebral catastrophe reflected on the reflex zones of the feet), solar plexus.
CRZ: Kidneys, heart, genitalia, intestine, cervical spine, neck and spleen.

ARM INJURIES
Zones on the feet: Cervical spine, shoulder girdle, shoulder joint, upper arm and elbow, teeth.

Consensual areas to be treated: Over the same area in the opposite arm, and 'energy-related' area, over the corresponding area of the leg which is the same side as the injured arm.

ARTHRITIS, ARTHROSES
Symptomatic zones: All joints, particularly those which are most affected; spine.
CRZ: Small intestine, large intestine, stomach, liver and gall-bladder, lymphatics — both upper and those of the pelvis; kidneys, adrenal glands, solar plexus, spleen, sinuses, teeth and scars.

AUTONOMIC DYSFUNCTION
Symptomatic zones: Solar plexus, head.
CRZ: Heart, endocrine system (particularly the pituitary gland and the genitalia) liver, intestine, kidneys, spine, shoulder girdle, sternum and spleen.
Graduate dosage with care and, in particular, conduct treatment mainly during expiration.

BED-WETTING
Symptomatic zones: Urinary tract, genitalia, lymphatics of the pelvis and inguinal canal.
CRZ: Lower spine, solar plexus, endocrine system; avoid strong geopathic irritations and unhealthy stimuli in the surroundings.

BREAST SWELLING AND TENDERNESS
Symptomatic zones: Breast and upper lymphatics.
CRZ: Shoulder girdle, genitalia, solar plexus, pelvic lymphatics and teeth.
If there is no improvement after the next menstrual period, the patient should be advised to seek specialist advice.

BRONCHIAL ASTHMA
Symptomatic zones: Respiratory tract, throat, upper lymphatics, diaphragm and sternum.
CRZ: Neck, occiput, shoulder girdle; all organs of the digestive tract, (particularly the small intestine and the ileo-caecal valve), the endocrine system (particularly the adrenal glands), the spleen, heart and spine.
When an acute attack threatens, firmly grip the webs between the second and third toes of both feet and massage the solar plexus reflex zone.

BRONCHITIS, BRONCHIECTASIS
Symptomatic zones: Respiratory tract, throat, upper lymphatics and diaphragm.
CRZ: Small intestine (particularly the ileo-caecal valve), large intestine, liver and gall-bladder, shoulder girdle, spleen, genitalia, urinary tract, heart.

'CERVICAL' SYNDROME
Symptomatic zones: Cervical spine, neck, shoulder girdle and head.
CRZ: Lower spine, solar plexus, teeth and correction of posture.

CHOLECYSTITIS
Symptomatic zones: Gall-bladder on both plantar and dorsal aspects, liver and small intestine, (particularly the duodenum).
CRZ: Right half of the shoulder girdle, solar plexus, (also that which angers and worries the patient), large intestine, pancreas and thoracic spine; attention to diet!
For colic: Use the sedation grip.

CONCUSSION
Symptomatic zones: All head zones, particularly the occiput and cervical spine.
CRZ: Solar plexus, heart, upper lymphatics, lower spine and stomach.

CONSTIPATION
Symptomatic zones: Large intestine (particularly the sigmoid, rectum and anus), liver, gall-bladder and small intestine (particularly the ileo-caecal valve).
CRZ: Pelvic lymphatics, lower spine, solar plexus, stomach, pancreas, head, endocrine system; investigate the dietary habits.

CYSTITIS, IRRITABLE BLADDER
Symptomatic zones: Bladder, ureter, kidneys.
CRZ: Lower spine, pelvic lymphatics, genitalia (particularly the prostate in male patients), spleen, solar plexus, pharynx and larynx, teeth.

DIABETES MELLITUS
This is supplementary treatment for patients in whom the blood sugar levels are controlled by drug administration. (Regular

assessment of blood sugar levels is necessary, especially in acute infections).
Symptomatic zone: Pancreas.
CRZ: Endocrine system, solar plexus (in shock diabetes), small intestine, large intestine, liver and gall-bladder, spleen, eyes and teeth.

DIAPHRAGM TREATMENT
Treatment of the reflex zone to the diaphragm should be included at least once in each massage. The more debilitated or disturbed the patient, the more frequently should this measure be included in your treatment. In between treating reflex zones which are painful, treat the diaphragmatic reflex zone following the inspiration and expiration of the patient. When the patient breathes in, apply gentle pressure to the reflex zone bimanually, at the same time flexing the feet towards the head. When the patient breathes out, gently rotate the feet outwardly to a position of light extension, and release the pressure on the reflex zone.

At the end of each massage, gently massage this area to sedate the patient, (the same zone as that for the solar plexus), and by paying attention to the personal respiratory rhythm of the patient bring the treatment session to a tranquil end.

DIARRHOEA
Symptomatic zones: Small intestine, pylorus and ileo-caecal valve.
CRZ: Solar plexus, liver and gall-bladder, large intestine, stomach, pancreas, endocrine system and middle spine.

EAR INFECTIONS
Symptomatic zones: Ears, lymphatics of the throat and pharynx.
CRZ: Teeth and sinuses, upper lymphatics, solar plexus, spleen, appendix, stomach and digestive tract.

EPILEPSY AND SIMILAR DISORDERS SUCH AS PETIT MAL
As supplementary therapy:
Symptomatic zones: Endocrine system, solar plexus, head and lymphatics.
CRZ: Spine, liver and gall-bladder, small and large intestines, spleen, scars, focus of infection.

FRACTURES
Symptomatic zones: Those zones which correspond to the injured tissues surrounding the fracture, lymphatics, solar plexus.
Fractures of the extremities: Consensual and 'energy-related' areas with the usual massage grip.

GLAUCOMA
Only as a supplementary measure when the patient is being seen by a specialist:
Symptomatic zones: Head, particularly the eyes, sinuses.
CRZ: Cervical spine, shoulder girdle, upper lymphatics, teeth and throat, kidneys, pancreas and solar plexus.

HALLUX VALGUS, CORNS, CALLOUSES
These are, in general, an outward indication that there is an inner taxation of the organ corresponding to the reflex zone over which the abnormality is located when persisting for more than a week. It indicates that treatment is required; a chiropodist should also be visited.

HAYFEVER
Symptomatic zones: Area of the nose and throat, sinuses.
CRZ: Upper lymphatics, liver, small intestine, (particularly the ileo-caecal valve), large intestine, bronchi, endocrine system, kidneys and spleen.

HEADACHE, MIGRAINE
Symptomatic zones: Head, (particularly the mastoid process), neck and cervical spine.
CRZ: Shoulder girdle, small and large intestines, stomach, liver and gall-bladder, spine, urinary tract, genitalia, (in women this is often associated with menstrual disorders), solar plexus, foci of infection; posture should be corrected if necessary.

HEART AND CIRCULATORY DISORDERS
The treatment is the same whether the origin of the disorder is stress or organic disease; the treatment may also be used as prophylaxis against infarction or treatment for recent or past myocardial infarction.
Symptomatic zones: Heart, left side of the shoulder girdle as far as the indirect reflex zone to the elbow, the sternum (which should be very gently treated immediately after an infarct).

CRZ: Diaphragm, upper lymphatics, liver and gall-bladder, stomach, small and large intestines, the diaphragm over the area where maximal stimulus is effected (because of the gastrocardial symptom complex); the cervical spine, (particularly the seventh cervical vertebra, and by very gently rotating the big toe on its base joint); the spleen, solar plexus, scars and teeth.
Remember that these patients often display a hypersensitivity to synthetically manufactured objects and fabrics!

HERNIA
Also postoperatively:
Symptomatic zones: Inguinal canal (particularly on the medial aspect related to the same body zone on the feet), pelvic lymphatics and genitalia.
CRZ: Lower spine, endocrine system (particularly the pituitary gland).

HYPERTENSION AND HYPOTENSION
Symptomatic zones: head, neck, heart and solar plexus.
CRZ: Shoulder girdle, kidneys, spine, digestive tract, foci (scars and teeth) and endocrine system.

JOINT DISORDERS
As well as massage of the symptomatic reflex zones and the causal reflex zones on the feet, consensual treatment of the joints may be given; i.e. if there is pain or disability of the shoulder joint, the opposite shoulder joint is treated, and if the ankle joint is painful and/or impaired in function, the opposite ankle is treated. The 'energy-related' joint may also be treated, so that when there is dysfunction of a hip joint, the shoulder joint on the same side of the body is treated, and similarly the hip joint on the same side of the body is treated where there is dysfunction of the shoulder joint. This allows treatment of:
knee joints for the elbow joints and vice versa;
joints of the hands for joints of the feet and vice versa;
treatment of the same joint on the opposite side of the body.
These areas are treated with the customary massage grip.

LEG INJURIES
Zones on the feet; Lower spine, pelvic region, hip and knee joints, teeth and sinus regions.
Consensual areas to be treated: Over the corresponding area on the

other leg, and in the 'energy-related' limb, that is over the corresponding area of the arm on the same side as the injured leg.

LYMPHATIC OBSTRUCTION DURING PREGNANCY
The first treatment should be very carefully and accurately dosed.
Symptomatic zones: Lymphatics of the pelvis and shoulder girdle, endocrine system.
CRZ: Heart, urinary tract, liver and gall-bladder, small intestine, large intestine (particularly the rectum and anus), solar plexus and spine.
The only contra-indication for treatment is when the pregnancy is unstable.

'MANAGER'S' ILLNESS
Symptomatic zones: Solar plexus, heart and sternum.
CRZ: Liver, small intestine, (particularly the duodenum), stomach, large intestine, endocrine system, spine and shoulder girdle.

MENISCUS INJURIES
May also be used as post-operative treatment:
Zones on the feet: All the reflex zones to the knee joints, lower spine, hip joint and pelvic region, pelvic lymphatics, teeth and scars.
Consensual areas to be treated: Treatment to the 'energy-related' zone may be given to the knee on the other leg, and the elbow of the arm on the same side as the injury or operation.

MENSTRUAL DISORDERS
Symptomatic zones: Pelvic lymphatics, genitalia and fallopian tubes.
CRZ: Endocrine system (particularly the pituitary and thyroid glands), lower spine, solar plexus, pelvic region and the indirect reflex zones to the thigh.
You should inform your female patients that menstruation may occur either earlier or later than expected, as reflex zone massage sometimes changes the cycle.

PERIPHEROVASCULAR DISEASE
Symptomatic zones: Lymphatics of the pelvis and the shoulder girdle, spine.

CRZ: Liver and gall-bladder, small and large intestines, solar plexus, endocrine system (particularly the pancreas), scars; attention should be given to consensual relationships!

PROSTATIC DISORDER
Also post-operatively:
Symptomatic zones: Genitalia and pelvic lymphatics
CRZ: Endocrine system, urinary system, lower spine, solar plexus, inguinal canal, throat and teeth.

RENAL DISEASE
Symptomatic zones: Kidneys, ureter and bladder.
CRZ: Lower spine, lymphatics of the pelvis and the inguinal region, spleen, heart, digestive tract, endocrine system, eyes, foci, (as yet inapparent disease, scars or chronic infections of an organ, or devitalized or impacted teeth).
For colic: Sedation grip

RHEUMATISM
Symptomatic zones: All joints which are painful, all organs and/or muscles which are painful.
CRZ: Small and large intestines, entire lymphatic system, spine, solar plexus, kidneys and adrenal glands, spleen, foci (teeth and scars); dietary habits and nutrition should be investigated.

SCIATICA, LUMBAGO
Symptomatic zones: lower spine, pelvic region.
CRZ: Kidneys, liver, intestine, pelvic lymphatics, genitalia, upper and lower spine, foci, solar plexus; correction of posture.

SINUSITIS
Symptomatic zones: All the sinus cavities of the head, the lymphatics of the face and throat (particularly the tonsils).
CRZ: Head, shoulder girdle, bronchi, spleen, small intestine (particularly the ileo-caecal valve), liver, pancreas, urinary system, genitalia.

SLEEP DISTURBANCES
Symptomatic zones: Solar plexus.
CRZ: Endocrine system (particularly the adrenal and pituitary glands), heart, spine, liver and gall-bladder, small intestine, large intestine and shoulder girdle, it may be necessary to change

dietary habits. Avoid geopathic irritations and radios, television and digital clocks in the bedroom.

STOMACH DISORDERS

Symptomatic zones: Stomach, cardia and pylorus.
CRZ: Solar plexus, middle spine, small intestine, (particularly the duodenum), large intestine, liver and gall-bladder, pancreas, endocrine system (particularly the pituitary gland), teeth and scars; dietary habits and lifestyle may need modification.

TOOTHACHE

As a first aid measure:
Use the sedation grip on the zone which corresponds to the afflicted tooth or teeth. Reflex zone massage is no substitute for the dentist!

Bleeding gums are an indication that metal which is antipathetic to the body has been used to fill the teeth or as a brace. Such metals should be removed and as yet subclinical disease should be treated. Nutrition should be improved.
Note: Although the teeth are essential for mastication and speech, they also, through the energy field which they share with the organs of the body in corresponding zones, are related to every organ.

TONSILLITIS

Also as post-operative treatment:
Symptomatic zones: Tonsils and lymphatics of the throat and neck.
CRZ: Entire lymphatic system, all head zones, spleen, cervical spine, shoulder girdle, ileo-caecal valve and appendix, digestive tract, liver, small intestine, heart.

THYROID DISORDERS

Symptomatic zones: Thyroid gland and the throat; commence treatment extremely gently when the patient has hyperthyroidism.
CRZ: Endocrine system, (in women particularly the ovaries), shoulder girdle, cervical spine, solar plexus, heart, lymphatics and teeth.

ULCUS CRURIS

Symptomatic zones: Lymphatics of the pelvis.

CRZ: liver, small intestine, large intestine, rectum, anus, urinary tract and endocrine system (particularly the pancreas); attention should be given to nutrition.

VARICOSE VEINS, PHLEBITIS

When the varicose veins are far advanced or infected the corresponding area on the arm of the same side of the body should be massaged. Thrombophlebitis is a contra-indication for reflex zone massage.

Symptomatic zones: Lymphatics of the pelvic region and liver.
CRZ: Small intestine, large intestine, (particularly the rectum and anus), heart, spleen, diaphragm and spine.

Bibliography

[1] Dicke, Elizabeth. *Meine Bindegewebsmassage*: Hippokrates Verlag, Stuttgart.

[2] Helmrich, Dr med. H. Die Bindegewebsmassage: Karl F. Haug Verlag, Heidelberg.

[3] Pschyrembel, Prof. Dr W. *Klinisches Wörterbuch*: Verlag Walter de Gruyter, Berlin.

[4] Ingham, Eunice D. *Stories the Feet Can Tell*:

[5] Ingham, Eunice D. *Stories the Feet Have Told*:

[6] Kneipp, Sebastian. *Meine Wasserkur*: Kösel-Verlag, Kempten.

[7] Mozer, Dr med. H. *Brennpunkte der Krankheiten*: Karl F. Haug Verlag, Heidelberg.

[8] Leboyer, Dr med. Frederic. *Birth Without Violence*: Fontana, 1977.

[9] Reckeweg, Dr med. H.H. *Homotoxinlehre*: Aurelia-Verlag, Baden-Baden.

[10] Voll, Dr med. R. *Topographic Positions of the Measurement Point in Electro-acupuncture*:

[11] Rauch, Dr med. E. *Die Darmreinigung nach F.X. Mayr*: Karl F. Haug Verlag, Heidelberg.

[12] Rauch, Dr med. E. *Blut- und Säfte-Reinigung*: Karl F. Haug Verlag, Heidelberg.

[13] Rosendorff, Dr med. *Neue Erkenntnisse aus der Naturheilbehandlung*: Turm-Verlag, Bietigheim.

[14] Namikoshi, T. *Shiatsu: Japanese Finger Pressure Therapy*: Japan Publications, 1973.

[15] Walb, Dr med. L. *Die Haysche Trenn-Kost*: Karl F. Haug Verlag, Heidelberg.

[16] Schaarschuh, Alice. *Atmungs- und Lösungstherapie bei Schlafstörungen*: Turm- Verlag, Bietigheim.

[17] Palm, Dr med. H. *Das gesunde Haus — unser nächster Umweltschutz*: Ordo-Verlag, Konstanz.

[18] Bressler, Harry Bond. *Zone Therapy*: Health Research, P.O. Box 70, Mokelumne Hill, California 95 245.

[19] Fitzgerald, William H. and Bowers, Edwin F. *Zone Therapy*: Health Research, P.O. Box 70, Mokelumne Hill, California 95 245.

[20] Mességué, Maurice. *Health Secrets of Plants and Herbs:* Collins, 1979.

[21] Reimkasten, Felix. *Die Alexander-Methode. Bedeutung, Folgen und Abstellung von Haltungsschäden*: Karl F. Haug Verlag, Heidelberg.

[22] Alexander, Gerda. *Eutonie*: Kösel-Verlag, München und Kempten.

Index